PSYCHIC MASSAGE

Roberta DeLong Miller

Photographer • Richard Tomlinson

Illustrator • George Armstrong

HARPER COLOPHON BOOKS
Harper & Row, Publishers
New York, Hagerstown, San Francisco, London

PSYCHIC MASSAGE

Copyright © 1975 by Roberta DeLong Miller. All rights reserved. Printed in the United States of America. No part of this book may be used or reproduced in any manner without written permission except in the case of brief quotations embodied in critical articles and reviews. For information address Harper & Row, Publishers, Inc., 10 East 53d Street, New York, N.Y. 10022. Published simultaneously in Canada by Fitzhenry & Whiteside Limited, Toronto.

First HARPER COLOPHON edition published 1975

LIBRARY OF CONGRESS CATALOG CARD NUMBER: 74–13477

STANDARD BOOK NUMBER: 06–090353–8

83 84 85 15 14 13 12 11 10 9 8

To Anne Armstrong, who taught me
that the body is a tool for spirit

CONTENTS

Introduction

This book describes a method of healing. It evolved from massage, yet it is more than massage. The addition of psychic awareness makes it possible to heal or balance a person's mind and emotions through his body.

Psychic massage cannot be learned by reading. It can only be learned by doing—very much like playing a musical instrument. Therefore, this book is organized in a "how to" format, so that those who wish may try out the techniques. My primary purpose, however, is to inform rather than to instruct—to present the possibilities and potentialities of a new approach to personal growth.

I

Self Preparation

To touch someone else you must be able to touch yourself. So close your eyes and take a moment to feel what you are like inside . . .

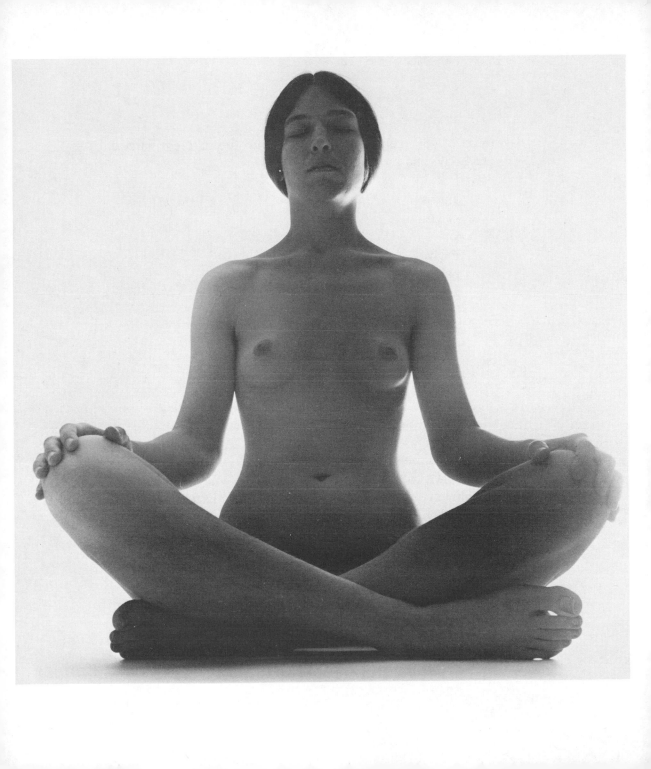

Put all of your conscious awareness into the different parts of
your body, one by one:

> feet
> ankles
> calves
> knees
> thighs
> pelvis
> genitals
> belly
> chest
> back
> shoulders
> arms
> hands
> neck
> head
> top of head

In each place you will probably experience yourself differently,
not only in terms of inner dimension but also in terms of emotional quality, color, tenseness, ability to feel.

Are you breathing?

Notice whether as you inhale everything expands—belly, ribs, chest, shoulders, back, pelvis—and as you exhale everything contracts. Breathe in, and the whole body goes out. Breathe out, and the whole body comes in.

As you breathe, explore inside your torso, neck, and head. Come to rest at the lowest place you feel comfortable. This is your center. If you can't find your center in your belly, about two fingers' width below the navel, look for it around your solar plexus or diaphragm.

Your center is the place where you are. Watch what happens there as you relax and breathe. I n h a l e . . . and E x h a l e. Something moves into center as you inhale, disperses from center as you exhale. First something is received, then something given.

Suppose you find your center just below the rib cage at the solar plexus. On the inhale, something like light or some magnetic force enters your body there. Exhale, and the force released rushes to all parts of your body—legs, feet, arms, hands, head—even outside your body. You become energized.

This may not happen immediately. You may need to practice feeling from your center. The sensations are subtle: vibration, tingling, magnetism, or rivulets of Energy flowing through and around you.

Your first experience of this Energy will probably be as magnetism or heat, rather than as a moving current.

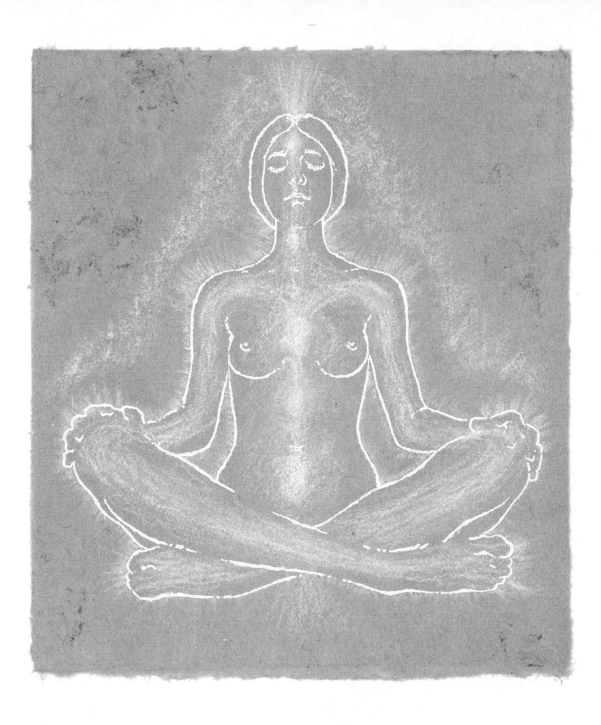

Become aware of your hands for a moment. If you place one palm facing the other about five inches apart, a magnetic field will build up after a few breaths. Notice that it takes effort to pull your hands apart. You must keep breathing. Otherwise the field collapses, your fingers, which were stiff with electricity, begin to wilt and curl up.

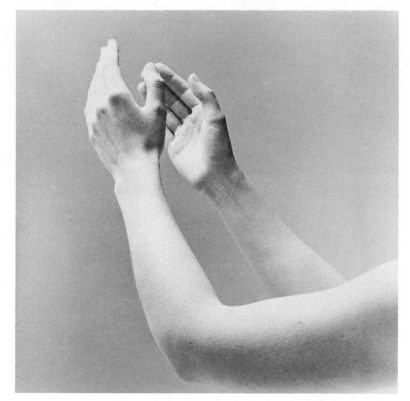

After you try this several times, the charge between your hands may begin to flow. In general, as you inhale you'll find Energy moving into your hands and through your arms into your center. As you exhale, the Energy reverses direction and goes out the arms and hands.

You may find Energy flowing outside the surface of your hands and arms. It is passing through invisible bodies which extend beyond the physical. Together, these bodies constitute your *aura*.

Ordinarily you cannot see your aura, but if you close your eyes, center yourself, and breathe, you will feel yourself expanding outwards. Your experience of self does not stop at the skin.

If you are having a hard time feeling Energy, try these exercises with a friend.

Sit facing one another. First, breathe in and out from your center several times. Get to know what you feel like apart from your friend. Then grasp your friend's hands and experience the difference from when you were alone. Joined, you should feel a higher level of bodily excitation or electrical current. Also, you may feel moved or touched inside by a quality which is your friend's rather than your own. With more practice, you may actually experience the current moving between you as a vibration, traveling in waves〜〜〜〜or pulsations⋀⋀⋀.

Next, have your friend sit quietly while you feel his aura. Follow the surface of his body with your hands two or three inches away from the skin. Start above his head; slowly go over his face and down his front. Also, check out the arms and hands, legs and feet. What do you feel? Heat . . . radiation . . . force . . . pushing away . . . letting in . . . prickling sensations . . . You'll probably have the strongest experience of Energy at the places indicated.

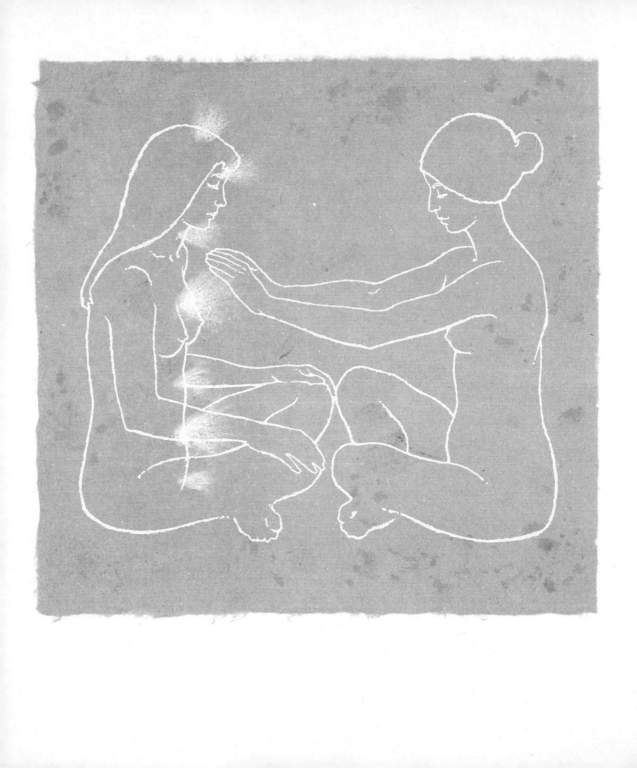

Come back to your own body again. If you found spots that radiated strongly in your friend, explore these in yourself. What happens in each place as you breathe? Do you feel a point of light getting bigger? Do you sense yourself making more space in your body around that point? Do you feel refreshed, revitalized there?

Now try something else by yourself. Stand up. Place your feet a few inches apart, toes pointing straight ahead. Bend your knees a little, so that your spine is comfortably erect.

As you inhale, imagine that there's a blue-white light moving in through the front of your belly, up your spine, and out the top of your head. As you exhale, the light moves from above the head, down the face, through the heart and visceral organs, and out the base of the torso.

    Inhale—Energy in through center, up the spine.

    Exhale—Energy down the front, out the base.

Try it ten to fifty breaths.

Still standing, relaxed, knees easy, place your hands in front of your belly.

Now pay attention to the movements of your body as you breathe. On the inhale, your belly fills and your pelvic bones move sideways to make room. Simultaneously, your rib cage expands. Your back widens. Air in the chest stretches your shoulders up and out. Hands separate to encompass more space. On the exhale, stomach comes in, pelvis narrows and drops under, chest recedes, hands touch again. Exaggerate the movement for awhile.

The tingling that moves down your legs and up your spine is Energy: the flow of life.

If you can feel it now, experiment with directing it where you will. Breathe it from your center into your hands, into your feet, into your eyes. Breathe it straight out from your belly.

Focus the Energy to make it more intense. You can do this by slowly, deliberately contracting the muscles in your abdomen on the exhale. It feels like you are pressing the inner force into a narrow, potent beam.

The principle is the same as that of light. When the rays of a beam are not focused, its illumination is fuzzy, diffused, weak. When its rays come together in a line or at a point, the light is strong, clearly defined, penetrating.

Once you know how to focus Energy within your body, you won't have to think about doing it anymore. The body will focus automatically as long as you stay inside the experience of channeling Energy.

The idea now is to relax your body as much as possible, so that it becomes totally receptive. You will feel your cells opening up, like flowers, in the presence of a cosmic sun.

Soon your awareness of Energy increases as you are able to allow more and more to move through you. I have experienced it at times as powerful rushes that start way above my head and travel to my feet in waves. At other times it feels like strength flowing out from my belly. You will find your own special way of knowing you've become a channel for the flow.

II

The Massage

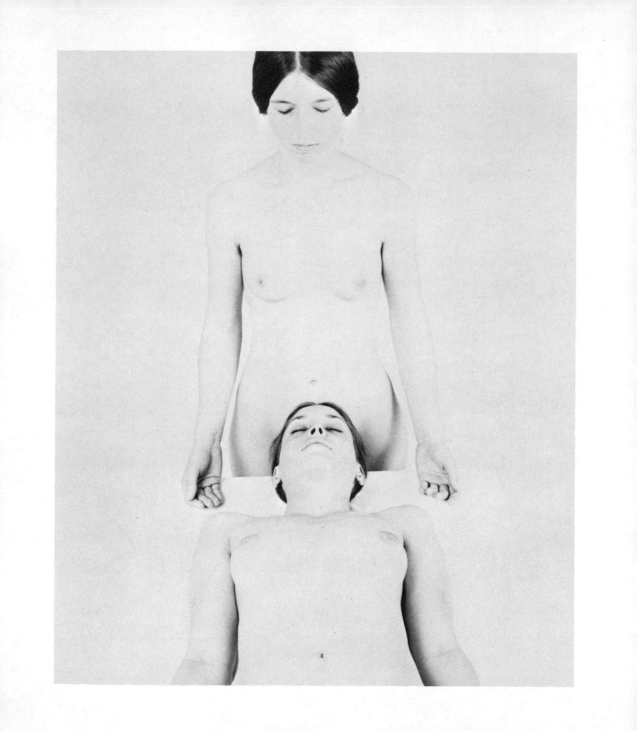

Now you are ready to begin working.

The person you will massage should be lying on his back before you, on a table as high as your hips.

Oil your hands, preferably with sesame oil. Then stand relaxed and open at the head of the table with your eyes closed. Feel the vibrations coming from the person. An Energy flow begins to circle from his aura through yours and back again. This is called making contact.

Contact is not made by reaching out with your physical body to another physical body. Rather, you reach someone by being within yourself and finding him there too. Contact is not between two but it is being one.

When you feel connected with the person, you may know intuitively which part of his body to touch first, which second, which last. Follow your feelings about what you want to do—they're usually right.

However, if you aren't sure how to proceed, you can begin by using the following massage as a pattern. It is a shortened form of the Esalen massage, designed to open the body's Energy channels. Don't worry about the precise way to perform the strokes. Where I feel it's important, I've included suggestions, but feel free to experiment on your own.

When Energy is flowing through your hands, they will transform
the person's body wherever they touch. The tissues are opened.
Tightness is replaced by a feeling of expansion, a sense of well-
being, a capacity for joy and pleasure. Feel these changes happening as you work over the large masses of the body. Begin with
the chest.

Very, very slowly and gently, place your hands on the person's chest. Slowly, let them sink in without pressing, until you feel more contact energetically. The flow will be stronger; you'll feel as though your hands are inside, rather than outside, his body.

As Energy circulates between you and the person, you'll notice that Energy is given and received simultaneously. At first, perhaps, it will seem that you're receiving as you inhale and giving as you exhale. But as your own body opens more and more to the life-force, you'll find that your giving is continuous and that you receive the other's unique vibration without interruption.

Slowly, push your palms and thumbs down the breastbone to the bottom of the rib cage, around to the sides of the torso, and up. Repeat several times. Then, run your fingers in between the ribs on both sides, with pressure in one direction, feather-light return. Massage directly under the collar bones with circular strokes. Then massage the pectoral muscles at the top of the chest.

Work in detail around the breastbone, and finally, let your hands rest over the heart center—just to the right of the heart. Breathe, and send Energy into this place. Make connection with the person's emotional being.

Then take your hands away, remembering to withdraw so slowly that the person can't be sure you're gone.

Though some teachers say your hands should never leave the body, I find that the person is refreshed by the chance to be with himself for a few moments.

After gathering more oil for your hands, repeat the first stroke on the chest (down the center, up the sides), and then continue it around the shoulders, under the upper back, up the neck, and under the back of the head. Let the total surface of your hands conform to the body contours as much as possible. Repeat several times. The person will surrender his head to your control if you hold it securely, then leave it slowly and gently. Encourage him to let go, so the Energy flows more freely.

Now focus your attention on the neck and shoulders. Think of them as double doors between the torso and the head. The doors are closed when the person doesn't want his feelings: he tightens his neck and shoulders to keep them subconscious.

To open those doors, first massage in egg-shaped circles just above the shoulder blades. Palms are facing upward as you work with your fingertips under the body. Rhythm is slow, pressure heavy, yet you must still be able to feel Energy contact. Start at the outer shoulders, press along the top of the shoulder blades (above the bone) toward the spine. Both hands approach the spine from opposite directions simultaneously. Go along the spine two inches toward the head, then back along the top of the shoulder. If you feel you can't exert enough pressure, kneel and do the same stroke with your thumbs; your fingers will be resting over the collar bones. Feel free to reverse the direction of the circular pathways.

Work next between the scapulae (shoulder blades) and the spine. Slip your hands underneath the back, palms up. You may want to leave your thumbs hooked over the shoulder. Explore in circles, using the sensitivity of your fingers to find out which muscles are holding tight. Push the scapulae away from the center of the body. Finally, loosen the connective tissue around and in between the thoracic vertebrae. Your goal is to free a channel through which Energy can be released upward.

If you've been successful in opening the shoulders, you will feel strong contact with the person at two places. The first is a small indentation on the upper edge of the shoulder blade. Hold your middle fingers in the two hollows, respectively, and allow four to ten breaths to establish connection with the organs inside the rib cage.

Then, gather your fingers together over the spine, just under the seventh cervical vertebra (the one that protrudes at the base of the neck) to test for Energy flow up the spinal column. If you feel a strong current coming into your hands, you'll know that you're enabling the person to connect consciously with what is going on in his depths.

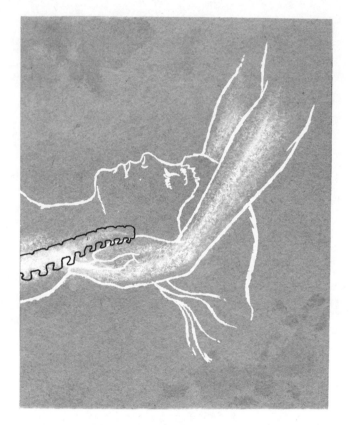

Now, extend your work into the neck by sliding your hands further up the spine—your fingers may cover it, but do not exert heavy pressure right on top of the bones. Massage carefully around each cervical (neck) vertebra, starting at the base of the neck and ending with the atlas, which supports the head. You'll probably find at least one vertebra embedded in a rigid mass of connective tissue, which stops the Energy flow between head and shoulders. It may also have an adverse effect on the person's voice, vision, or hearing. Give that vertebra extra time and attention.

Now, putting your palm above one ear, turn the person's head to that same side, resting his forehead against your forearm. Massage the neck with your free hand. Some of your strokes should move all the way out to the edge of the shoulder and return. Give special care to the muscles just under the bony ridge of the skull—massage in small circles from spine to ear.

Then you will want to scratch the person's scalp with the fleshy part of your fingertips, actually moving the skin over the cranium. Work over the upturned half of the scalp twice, releasing tension behind the ear and at the temple. Then, place your palm over the crown, or perhaps an inch away, to see whether Energy is flowing now up through the head, as it should if the body is to experience full vitality.

Turn the head to the other side and repeat.

Centering the head again, cup your hands on either side of the skull. Gently but firmly stretch the neck, using your body like a sandbag weight, until you feel the vertebrae in the spinal column releasing Energy upward, one by one.

Without breaking continuity, move to the face. The face, like all other parts of the body, is flesh and bone, so don't be afraid to work deeply. Use no additional oil.

Generally, the face is massaged from the midline outward—for example, when you smoothe muscles on the forehead, or over and under the brow, you should end your strokes at the temples. Work carefully over the cheeks to the jaw muscles, where you will probably use a lot of pressure and still not loosen them enough. Encourage the person nonverbally to let his jaw hang open, lips and teeth parting. Attend to the stiff upper lip, the cleft of the chin, and muscles under the jaw bone. For the last, put your thumbs over the top of the chin and fingers just inside the bone underneath; stroke firmly all the way around the back of the jaw to the ear lobes.

Finally, place your fingers over the "third eye"—between, and a little above, the person's eyebrows. You will be contacting, and hopefully strengthening, the intuitive faculty. Feel whether there is an Energy flow connecting the third eye with the rest of the body before you gently take your leave.

Next the arms.

But first, recenter yourself. Become aware of your own breathing again and of the flow in, through, and around your own body.

Move to the person's right side. Stand next to his hip, facing his head. Then put both hands on his right arm at the shoulder, and slowly spread oil down to his fingertips. Include his palm.

Put more oil on your hands. Facing the person's head, take his right wrist in your left hand; place your right palm on the inside of his forearm, and push it up toward the armpit as you walk forward with the arm and turn your own body half-circle clockwise. Your right hand continues its stroke over the person's chest to his hip, then up his right side and right arm to the elbow. You are now facing the torso, and the person's arm is extended over his head.

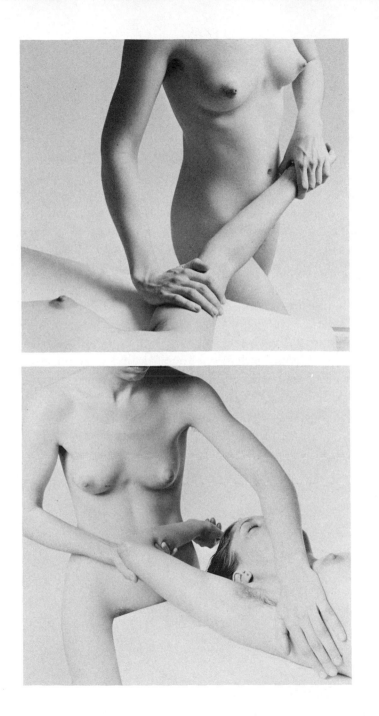

Give the elbow to your right hand. Then, spread the excess oil from your left hand over the inside of his right upper arm and torso. Return his elbow to your left hand and rest his forearm against your abdomen or hip for security. Massage the inside of the upper arm, still extended, with your right hand. Press your thumb on top as you go from his elbow to his shoulder and on the side as you return from shoulder to elbow. Your right wrist will be rotating.

With your right hand, work the muscles under the armpit, next to the shoulder blade. Bring both of your hands along the person's arm all the way to his wrist and stretch the arm overhead. Then, with your left hand holding the elbow and your right hand the wrist, walk toward the body and turn yourself back around to rest the person's elbow on the table. Keep his forearm raised.

With your left hand, massage the upper arm with long strokes and large circular strokes. Pay special attention to the hollows at the shoulder joint and the muscles just above the elbow.

Massage the person's forearm with long strokes moving away from the wrist. Your thumb will be pressing on one side, fingers on the other. Lift the forearm until it is vertical and the entire arm is off the table. Grip it loosely near the elbow with your palms while your fingers interlace, and let it slide to the table by means of its own weight.

Massage the back of the person's hand, still upright, by pressing your thumbs in between the tendons. Then, turn so that you face his palm. Press your thumbs from the base of the palm to each finger individually. Tension may be released from the fleshy area just under the fingers. Massage in circles.

Now, let the hand drop so that you are holding it in your right hand near the table, fingers pointing toward you. With your left thumb and index finger, pull gently and slowly on the person's little finger, then return and pull again; finish by turning round the tip of the finger as if you were following the grooves on a cork-screw. Do three fingers with your left hand and the remaining two with your right.

Then, lay the arm to rest at the person's side and bring it all together by stroking repeatedly from shoulder to hand—slowly enough to feel Energy exchange with every square inch of flesh you touch. Finally, just barely touching the arm, stroke lightly with the tips of your fingers.

As you finish, hold the person's hand between your own. You should experience Energy coming from the person's center through his arm, so that his center is touching your center by way of the hands.

Withdraw your hands slowly, and give the person a chance to sigh before you begin the same work on his left arm.

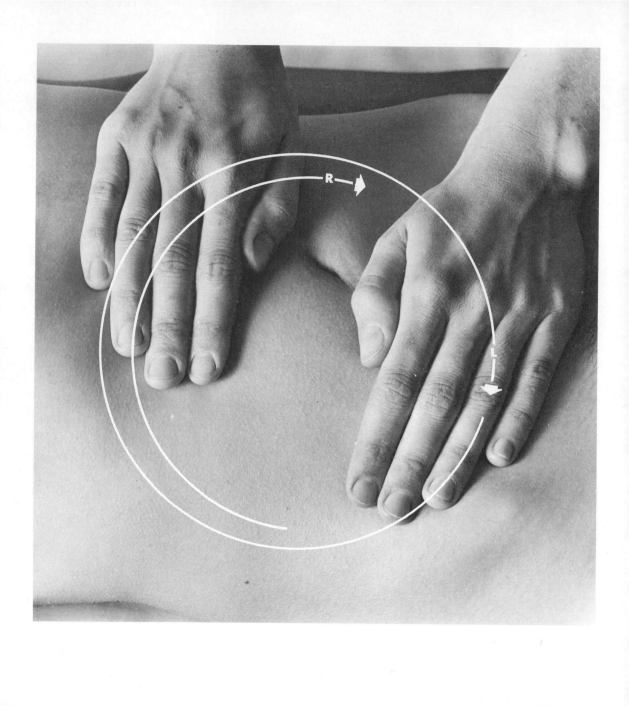

Having completed the arms, proceed to the abdomen.

Stand beside the person's waist. Rather than dropping your hands directly onto his stomach—it may frighten him—begin on his chest, which you've already massaged. As you slide your hands from the chest onto the abdomen, you'll begin massaging in a clockwise circular motion. This is tricky until you get the feel of it: left hand makes a full circle over the abdomen, right hand makes a half circle. Begin with the right hand at the far side of the body as the left hand passes the near side; come off the body at the near side as the left hand passes the far side. After you master that, let your hands follow the dips between the rib cage and the pelvis as they travel to the edge of the waist; the circle becomes elongated at the sides of the body. Besides being beautiful, this stroke has a particular advantage: the person cannot follow it with his brain. Rather than understanding what you're doing, he now has to experience it. He has to move his center of awareness out of his head and into his abdomen, where you want it to be.

Next, move your hands upward toward the rib cage to massage the diaphragm. Your upper hand is placed over the lower end of the breastbone. It should feel connected with your lower hand, which massages under the far side of the rib cage in a spiral beginning at the center of the body. After five or six loops pressing away from yourself and arriving under the lowest ribs, pull with a single stroke across the diaphragm from the far side of the body to your starting point.

Remember, as usual, to breathe in Energy.

Keeping one hand on the breastbone, walk around the person's head to the other side of his body, and repeat on the other half of the diaphragm.

Let your hands slide to the lower abdominal area. Move your body so that you are standing beside the person's thigh, facing his head. With your fingers together, push upwards along each side of the body's midline. You are massaging two long muscles called the *rectus abdominus*. Stroke upward with your fingers and thumbs several times; as you circle around, your hands go under the rib cage, down the sides of the body, and back to the midline above the pubic bone. You're drawing the picture of a butterfly.

There's another stroke you can do only if the person's stomach is loose. Place your hands side by side on the abdomen. Press down and toward the midline with your palms only . . . and lift up. Then from the other side press down and toward the midline with your fingers only . . . and lift up. Do this several times, finally moving the intestines almost circularly (clockwise) with this pressing from side to side. Again, a note of warning: this can cause pain if the belly is too tight.

Finally, place your hands directly over center (one and a half inches below the navel) and wait for contact with the person there. You must breathe Energy in and out and listen very sensitively for whatever connection is possible.

If the person is unable to give and receive at his belly center, you will experience deadness and a complete lack of vitality; in fact, you may want to take your hands away because you sense the person's fear of opening too much.

If, however, you are able to contact the person here, it can be a wondrous and awe-inspiring experience for both of you. The person's belly is his source of power and creativity when he is open and responsive to the life which is All Being. As your beam of Energy comes into that place, there is a synergetic gain of presence. No longer are you two bodies, but one overwhelming unity.

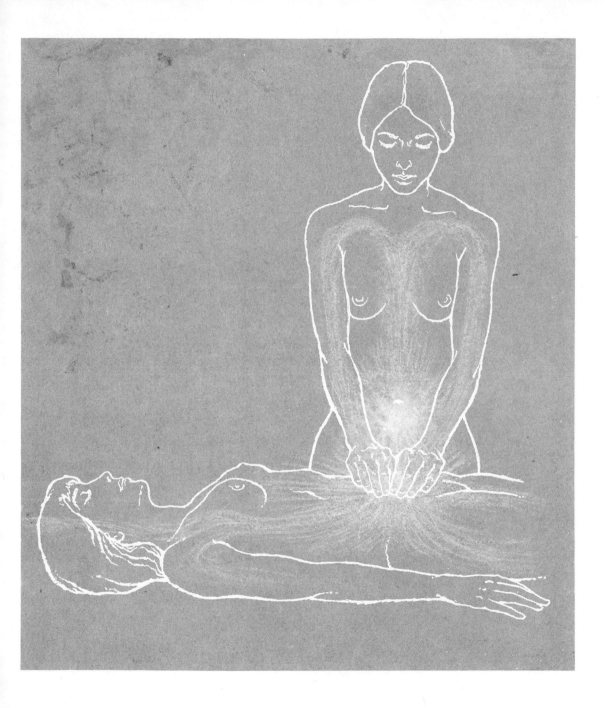

Come away from the belly by stroking lightly down both legs to the feet. Let this be the first indication to the person that his legs join his belly to the earth. They are his grounders.

Stand at the foot of the table. Put more oil on your hands, and begin stroking both legs upward from the feet. Turn from the inside to the outside of the thighs at the hip joint, and slowly stroke in the reverse direction all the way to the feet. This can be done many times, and it begins to feel better and better as the legs get used to accepting touch.

Connect the person's legs to his torso in whatever way feels comfortable. As an example, both hands could go up the right leg, up the right hip and ribs, around the shoulder, and down the right arm to the fingertips. Essentially, you're looking for strokes that cover the whole body.

Choose one leg, and after it is sufficiently oiled by full-length strokes, begin working with the thigh. Starting just above the knee, pull upward on the adductor muscles, moving up the inside of the thigh by alternating your hands. The last pull continues up over the groin. Then your hands begin again alternately pressing upward on the outside of the thigh from the hip to the knee.

Standing beside the knee, stroke up the center of the thigh with your palms or thumbs. The leg may tell you to move in half-circles as you do this. Probe for tension just above the knee.

Then massage around the outside of the kneecap. You can push it back and forth, since it floats on a bed of soft tissue. Press fairly deeply into the two depressions just below the kneecap—Energy gets held up there. With your fingers touching ever so lightly below the knee, begin a stroke that goes all the way down the calf to the ankle.

It's hard to massage the calf well from the front. Instead, try pressing the flesh sideways against the shinbone. For instance, you can stand beside the leg and cover the calf with both hands as though you were going to pinch it, fingers on the inside, thumbs on the outside. As you pull upwards, thumbs and fingers press to make new moon crescents.

You can also massage the calf lengthwise when you stand at the foot of the table. Squeeze the flesh of the calf with your palms, one hand on either side of the leg, fingers meeting underneath. It's good to do several long upward strokes just outside the shinbone, where the muscles tend to become stuck together.

Massage the front of the ankle with your thumbs, detailing the ligaments. Move around to the back of the anklebones with your fingers, and push the flesh upward to the point where the leg rests on the table.

Massage the top of the foot, first in circle-arc strokes with your thumbs, then with fingers moving in between the tendons. Search out the delicate indentations under the anklebone and around the heel. Massage the toes individually, moving each one in little circles. Slide a finger into the valleys between, and massage the base of each toe as well as the tip.

Now that you have completed all parts of the leg, connect them with long strokes as at the beginning. Cover the full length of the leg at least three times, then pass one or both of your hands over the person's stomach and down his other leg to the foot. Massage his other leg in the same way.

Then hold both feet. Tune in. If you've really opened the person's body, you will feel connected with all his parts through this one point of contact. Energy will be flowing from your hands up through his legs, torso, arms, and head, then back again. You will experience the person as translucent, glowing, vibrating with a trans-personal quality of love.

You will continue to feel the same connection even after you withdraw your hands one inch from the feet. Tarry there until you feel finished.

After the person rests long enough to savor his experience, ask him to turn over. Quietly place rolled towels under his ankles so that his legs are comfortable.

Then stand beside the person's waistline. Center yourself, as at the beginning. Again make contact with the person by experiencing him inside your extended self. Reluctantly, but surely, let your hands move through his aura to find a resting place at the small of his back. Give yourself lots of time to experience the person . . . all the way through his body to the front side, upward into his chest and head, downward into his legs and feet.

Spread oil sensitively over the person's back and legs, so that you won't need to do this later on. Use long strokes that cover the whole body (including the neck and arms).

When you actually begin the detailed work on the person's back-side, you will want to start at the feet and push Energy *up* the back in the same way you have already pushed it *down* the front.

Standing at the foot of the table, choose one leg, and after you have outlined its shape and quality with the usual long strokes, lift the calf off the table so that you can attend to the sole of the foot.

First, massage the arch with your thumbs alternately pressing from front to back. Then, while you hold the foot with one hand, work the heel with the other, squeezing it between your thumb, palm, and fingers. Massage in circles around the edge of the heel. Apply pressure to the ball of the foot with one thumb or both. Start under the toes and press the flesh away from you. This has the effect of straightening out the toes. Massage very carefully around the base of the toes.

Lay the foot back down on its towel. Massage the person's calf, then his thigh, with strokes that go up the center and down the sides. Use the same pulling and pinching techniques as you used for the front of the leg.

Include the buttock. Make sweeping movements that encircle the flesh. Then, with your thumbs moving alternately in strips from thigh to waist, check for tight places. Press the flesh up from the table with your palms; then pull it away from the midline as you work in very small circles beside the sacral vertebrae and the coccyx (tailbone). Hold two fingers under the tailbone while you make space between the pelvic bones and the spine with your other hand.

Proceed similarly on the other leg.

Connect both the person's legs with long strokes from the waist. Then, beginning at the heels, sweep all the way up his backside, over his shoulders, and down his arms. Without breaking continuity, begin work at the small of his back.

Reaching across to the opposite side of the person's body, pull your hands alternately up along the top of his pelvis to his spine. Continue the strokes either up or down the spine a few inches, and then return to the side of the body. You will be making elongated circles, which can be interrupted if both hands are going the same direction along the spine.

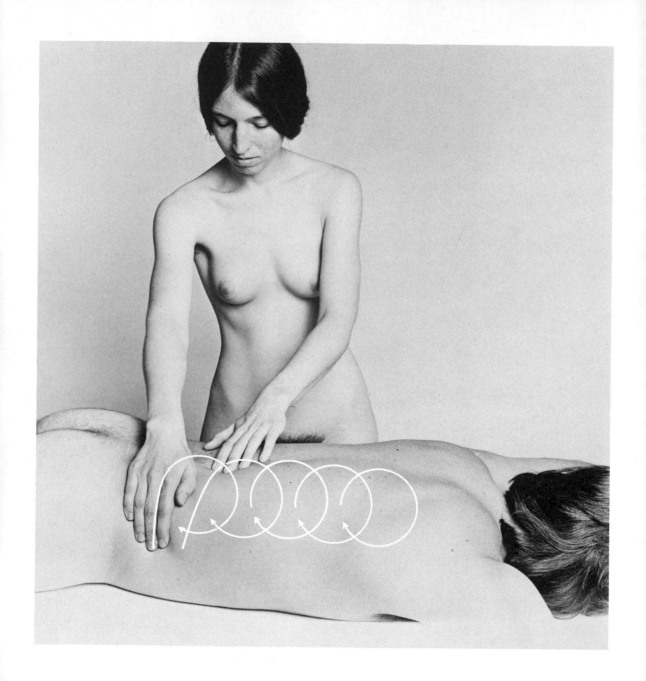

Continue the same pattern of stroking up the entire side of the back. One hand will be making full circles, the other half circles. Pressure should be used when you pull from the side of the body to the center and then move upward along the spine. And when you use pressure you should be exhaling, sending Energy into the body.

When you reach the top of that side of the back, hold one hand on the spine and walk around the person's head to the other side of his body. Repeat the entire sequence, starting by pulling just above the pelvic bone.

Now you have loosened the person's back generally. Your ultimate goal is to open his spine, which conducts Energy vertically in his body. However, you'll be most successful if you approach this in stages. The body needs time to open.

Place one hand at the base of the spine. Use your other hand to massage the *erector spinae* on the half of the back nearest you. This is a muscle grouping which extends the length of the back like a thick band, perhaps an inch from the vertebrae. Massage in circles from the top of the back downward, using either your fingers or the bony projection at the base of your palm, directly beneath your little finger. When you get to the bottom of the spine, use both hands alternately to push the flesh on that entire side of the back upward until you reach the shoulder blade.

Massage around and on top of the shoulder blade. Sometimes it helps to bring the person's hand, palm up, onto the small of his back. If the person's shoulder is too tight to allow this, simply place your forearm under his shoulder to lift the blade. In massaging around the shoulder blade, don't forget the ribs under the armpit.

Return the arm gently to the person's side. Walk around the body, and repeat the whole procedure on the other half of the back, beginning with the erector muscle.

Now, standing at the person's head, knead the top of the back
—trapezius, rhomboid muscles. Press with your palms; push the
shoulder blades away from neck and spine. Work the flesh between your fingers and thumbs.

Now you have come to the most important part of the massage. Move to one side of the body and begin investigating the vertebrae one by one, starting at the tailbone. Isolate them with your fingers. Massage around each one, loosening the connective tissue. Never press directly on the bone—press into the hollow between it and the next one. There may not be gaps between the lowest vertebrae. In an adult body they are often fused.

As you explore the person's spine, stop from time to time on vertebrae that arouse your curiosity. These may be bones that have an exceptionally strong current flowing out, or bones that feel almost dead, or bones that are out of line—too far left, too far right, too close to the neighboring vertebrae above or below. Because the vertebrae pass nerves to and from internal organs and tissues, when you touch one of these bones with Energy, changes begin to take place inside the body. If there is too much or too little Energy in a particular portion of the body, the imbalance also appears in the spine and can be corrected by your touch.

Now you will understand why the spine is so important. Each bone is an Energy access way into the body. When you have worked over the whole spine, you have massaged the entire body internally.

As well as stimulating a cross-sectional Energy flow by massaging the vertebrae individually, you will also want to check the Energy connection up and down the spine. Wherever you find a break in that connection (a displaced vertebra, for instance), spend more time there manipulating the tissues. Your goal is to help Energy flow from the top of the head downward and from the bottom of the feet upward through the spine, to create a balance between the two directions.

Now the massage is technically complete, but you may wish to cover the back again with playful or artistic touches. For example, you can draw figure eights on the halves of the back; you can massage in huge circles with your forearms; you can rake your fingernails gently from buttocks to shoulders.

To finish, re-focus your Energy to maximum intensity. Then, standing at the person's head, bend over and touch the base of his spine with all your fingers. Hold quietly until the person is totally with you at that spot. Then, draw your hands up the spine so slowly that the person stays with you all the way. Let his presence determine your speed. It should take you at least two minutes to travel from his coccyx to his head, drawing his Energy upward as you go.

The person will feel you moving his entire being, from his depths to his heights. His body begins to vibrate under your hands, like a sympathetic string harmonizing with you. The experience is overpowering.

After you reach his head, hold it a moment. You should be able to feel contact with the person all the way down to his toes. Then, let your hands draw back an inch. Because of continuing Energy exchange, the person will still feel touched all over. Withdraw your hands at least six inches from his head, or even further, to encompass his aura. Then, with blessing and thanksgiving, make your final departure.

III

Energy

Hopefully, Energy is flowing by now in your body and in the other person's body. This is what you have been trying to accomplish. Now it is time to understand in a more theoretical way what this Energy is like and how it is related to the way you experience yourself.

When you hold your hands a few inches apart, palm facing palm, you create a magnetic field between them. This magnetism indicates the presence of polarities, opposite poles which attract one another.

The first thing we can say about Energy is that it is composed of opposites. The best way to understand these opposites is to think of them as directions of force:

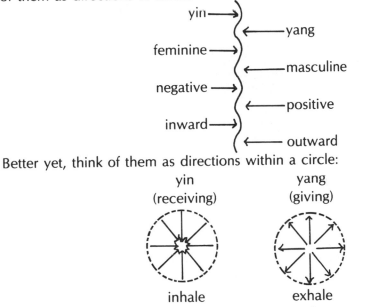

Better yet, think of them as directions within a circle:

yin   yang
(receiving)   (giving)

inhale   exhale

You may recall this experience in your center when you were breathing.

Though we divide them to talk about them, these opposites within Energy can never really be separated. One cannot exist without the other. Positive and negative pulls are both necessary for movement. This is what the Eastern philosophers were trying to say with their symbol for yin and yang. Together, the two create vibration.

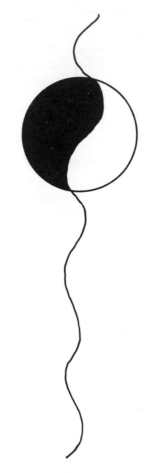

When the opposites are in correct relationship, the result is balance. Balance is the state of equilibrium, of satisfaction, of completion. If you have a need and it is filled, you are satisfied.

The second thing we can say about Energy is that it is balanced. Balance is the essence of health and life. Balance is the natural state of the universe.

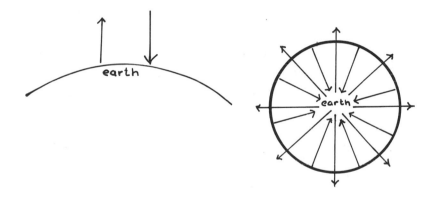

Now, despite the balanced quality of Energy, the human body can become unbalanced. As you looked inside your body for a center earlier, you may have noticed places that felt dark, heavy, and inert, rather than satisfied, complete, and loving. The darkness means that the movement of Energy has been interrupted.

These dark places exist because you, as a human being, have the power of choice. You can choose one vibration out of the total flow, and keep it, cherish it, imprison it, not let it dissolve back into the totality of things.

I'll refer to a single vibration you've separated out from Energy as *energy* with a lower-case *e*. Withheld energy can still vibrate, it still has electrical charge. On the other hand, it is limited, defined. It is held up, or holed up, inside the body so that it cannot be re-absorbed into Energy.

Since energies are by definition unbalanced, they have either positive or negative charges. Fear, sadness, revenge, self-pity, resentment are examples of negative energies. These feelings indicate that an inward force has been frozen; the person holds a loss, a lack, an emptiness. On the other hand, self-righteousness, pride, willfulness, possessiveness, piety are withheld positive energies. The person refuses to balance an outward thrust with corresponding negative forces. It takes sensitivity on your part to distinguish the joy that comes with fulfillment or balance from positive feelings that are stuck and unmoving.

Because they are incomplete forms of the universal Love or Logos, energies always set up a separation between one part of the whole and another part. They individuate *you* from *them* so that there is no longer a unity.

This separation manifests itself physically as well as psychologically. Held energies must occupy definable physical territories. You may have noticed this in yourself: perhaps you found sadness compacted near your heart, fear compressed in your belly. Locations are unique to each individual. Places that hold energies are separated as if by a wall from the natural flow in the rest of the body.

Whenever an energy occupies space in the flesh, no other vibration can pass through. Therefore, when you hold energies, your body's total capacity for channeling Energy is diminished.

Also, you experience yourself as emotionally heavy. This can be explained by the fact that you're holding something inside, rather than being an empty vessel continually refilled.

The presence of energies can manifest itself as physical weightiness as well. There is a connection between being physiologically clogged and emotionally immovable.

Another word for withheld energy would be *ego*. As I will use the term, ego refers to self-identity derived from energies contained or confined inside the body. Subconsciously, the person with an ego attachment begins to feel: "My self depends on holding this energy in me." "I'm real because I'm heavy; I have ballast." "I exist because I'm holding sadness, grief, rage."

Of course, this is an illusion, but a powerful one. Ego is powerful. When a person is heavy, when he has invested in the game of trapping energies, he isn't always attracted by the alternative of lightness, of fluidity, of ecstasy.

Believe it or not, you hold energies inside your body because you *want to,* and for no other reason. The positive or negative charge of an energy makes you feel something, though in fact the feeling is not always pleasant. You don't want to let go of that particular charge because you're used to it; it constitutes part of your view of the way things really are. The ego's fear is that if you let go of that feeling, you would no longer exist; there would be nothing to fill the space it occupied.

In truth, there is no void. Voidness is itself an ego energy. When the ego dies, or is emptied, cosmic Energy appears.

The very first step in clearing yourself—emptying your body of its energy contents—is to take responsibility for your own feelings, to admit that you like being unhappy, disappointed, angry, sad. Otherwise you wouldn't be that way.

Once you take response-ability for your feeling or thought, you will realize that you have the power to change that response if you wish. Given that you have a choice, you may decide to opt for a thought or feeling that makes you one with, rather than separate from, the rest of the universe. Only when you realize you no longer need ego energy to integrate your psyche can the energy be discharged.

Look into your body now to search for caught energy spaces. First, you will experience these as dead. The clogged energy at a certain location is not lively. It feels dark, heavy, inert. If you stimulate it—by attending to it inwardly and by sending it light—it may become active enough for you to feel. This does not mean it is free to leave its location, only that you are now aware of its qualitative identity. You know what feeling or thought it is that you have harbored.

Suppose you find anger in your belly. To discharge it, first *feel* the anger, experience its particular quality. Then, immerse yourself in it, let yourself be swallowed up by it. If it is protected by fear or resistance, experience or feel those energies too. You can find sentences, sounds, or movements to express the feeling, though once the feeling is flowing, you probably won't need them. Let the feeling spread over your entire body, particularly the extremities, because these are exit routes. You will experience streamings, vibration, or trembling as the energy that constitutes the feeling passes out of your body. And then in its place you may experience joy, contentment, peace.

Now that you've discharged the energy, be careful not to slip back into old habits. Ego power can be very seductive. You still make the choices. You may be accustomed to responding to certain situations with anger. Learn to slip out of that state of mind and into a forgiving or grace-full state of mind. It feels like turning the channel of an inner TV set. In any situation you have the choice of responding with acceptance or with rejection—making yourself one with someone or something, or making yourself separate.

The reason for describing this procedure in such detail is that your own sense of clarity is vital for the psychic work that follows. You cannot indulge in energies that create separation—anger, fear, control—while you are healing people. Instead, you must allow the Energy or life-force to move within you; then attunement is assured.

How do you know you're in the flow?

There is a sense of everything being as it should be: just right—in fact, *perfect.* If nothing needs to be different than it is, you don't have to judge or make things better. You can rest; a feeling of calmness and peace can sweep through your awareness.

When you touch someone, you will balance the forces around that person's body. You fill that which is depleted, you trim that which is superfluous, simply by your presence. And the longer you touch, the more the edges of the person's vibrations become smooth, the more the cacophonous sounds of his body become harmonious.

And when you work, the Energy moves you. In effect, it tells you what to do. There is no intellectual decision or thought about what is needed. You simply step into the river and go where it takes you.

100

And . . .

LOVE

. . . is the river's name.

IV

Healing Techniques

Energy is the source of all life. Yet, we interrupt that life within ourselves by grabbing pieces of the total Energy, which, alone, are unbalanced. Balance can be restored if we give up the caches of energy that obstruct it. This, very simply, is the process of healing.

Once you have experienced healing within yourself, you will better understand how it happens to the person you massage. The purpose of this chapter, then, is to provide specific instructions for helping the person's energies discharge, so that he can become more alive.

It is important to emphasize two things before proceeding with the instructions.

First, the process of healing takes time, since it occurs within the person at many levels of his being. You won't know whether you're massaging him at the beginning of his healing cycle or at the end. If you encounter him at the beginning, it may appear that not much is happening; actually the Energy from your hands smooths his overall vibration so the life within him gains the potency to move energies out at some later time. On the other hand, if you touch him at the moment he's ready to discharge, miracles may occur, but you'll have to give credit to other forces that previously set the whole process in motion.

Second, you can never do anything to another person. You simply make Energy available to him in a form he can use *if he chooses.* Ultimately, the responsibility for change rests with the person himself.

This leaves you free to give all the Energy you wish. The person will not take in more than he can handle. Let it be all right if the person cannot receive everything you know is available to him.

Now you are ready to study four principles of healing:
   General transference
   Structural correction
   Seeing
   Psychic reading
These are presented in order of their difficulty, so you should master the first before you try the second, and so on. For the purpose of instruction, the techniques are defined here separately and illustrated on parts of the body where they are easy to practice. Eventually, you'll use them all together, without differentiation, wherever you happen to be massaging.

Already you have found Energy flowing through your own body. However, you have also discovered places in your body that cannot pass the flow because they are choked up with lesser energies.

These same phenomena will be noticeable in the person you massage. As you explore his body, you'll find it is not equally open everywhere. Some places you touch feel alive, some feel dead. The former are flowing Energy, the latter are holding energies. Your hands will sense the difference. Where there is life, the Energy feels present, direct, centered, complete, timeless— you can connect with it in the *now*. Where there is ego, the energy has a limited, specific quality and a temporal duration— it started in the past and continues through time until it discharges in the future; you feel it as a series of pulsations that you cannot connect with, or get a hold of, in the present.

Life: now

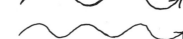

ego: duration through time

Fortunately, life has the power to move caught energy. If you breathe life through your hands into a dead space long enough, it will begin to respond directly. The response will be the specific energy content of that space. That is, if you breathe Life into an angry place, it will eventually respond with anger; if you activate a fearful spot, fear will emerge. When the old energy passes from the body, there is room for life to flow in its place.

I call this the principle of general transference. If you give a person life—love—Energy—he uses it to activate what is within and thus to become free.

First Principle: General Transference

So when you work with a great amount of Energy flowing in your own body, the body beneath your hands will surprise you with its responses. These may be emotional, physical, verbal or non-verbal. Some of the more dramatic ones are crying, laughing, screaming, moaning, shaking, pounding, coughing, yawning, vibrating, rocking, singing.

But don't let your attention be distracted by these. You're not interested in the form of expression pent-up energy uses, but in the energy itself. A person may cry forever, but if he doesn't let go of that which causes his tears, he will have to cry again. So, you're looking for the sadness that feels like flashes of electricity passing out of the person and through you, making your body zing and tingle. Then you know the work has been done.

Here is a typical example. I am massaging a man's face. Quite unexpectedly he grows restless, then agitated; he begins to growl or snarl and to press the table with his fists, while a few tears of rage escape over his temples. Yet, in all this activity I feel no current of energy release. Conclusion: nothing is happening yet. I gently hold my hands on that same spot a while longer. He appears to calm down. He takes a big breath, which tells me he is about to risk a change. Silently, without any demonstration, he looses a flood of anger and fear energy that quite overwhelms me. It feels like a wind passing through my aura in waves.

Of course, it's not always easy to get such a response. So you need more hints about how to let energy loose through general transference.

First of all, listen with your center for the readiness of a place to discharge energy. You'll find that not all dead places are equally inactive. In some the energy is dormant, but in others it is vibrating in place, or active. To save yourself time and Energy drain, you'll want to concentrate on the tissues that contain active ego energy that is just starting to come out to you.

For example, suppose as you're working on the person's chest, you feel irregular, jerky beats coming to you from the area of the breastbone, while the pectoral muscles give off no perceptible pulsations. The breastbone is ready to release energy, the pectorals aren't. This doesn't mean you wouldn't massage the pectorals —they may want and need manipulation—but it means you would listen more carefully to the breastbone where you felt a few beeps of vibrational rhythm. Then, you would work in small circles, or simply hold your hands there quietly, breathing life-force into the body and allowing its excess energy to flow through you. Soon what appeared to be a trickle of energy becomes a flood. It gushes out and is gone. Then the person is able to feel, to give and receive more than he imagined possible.

Second, use both of your hands on the body wherever possible. You are like a battery: your right hand is your positive pole, your left hand is your negative pole, and Energy travels between them. If one hand isn't connected to the person you're massaging, you'll have an incomplete circuit.

Finally, your body must act as a grounding pole for whatever comes in to you from the person. It's important to let his energies flow all the way through your arms, torso, legs, and feet into the floor or preferably the earth. Some of the energy you receive may be toxic. If you block it in your own body, it can cause you to feel ill or prevent your own good Energy from circulating freely. So ground it. Consciously open a channel to your feet through which unbalanced vibrations may be discarded.

General transference is the first and most basic principle of psychic massage. Passing Energy is the means by which you make contact; it is the manner in which you become the same as another person and can therefore know him; it is the method of restoring balance to his body.

The other three healing skills depend on this one for their effectiveness.

To understand the second principle of healing, you need to see that the physical body has mechanisms for keeping energies locked in.

When massaging the person's neck, you might check the location of his cervical vertebrae with your fingers. It's likely that at least one is out of line. It may be pulled inward toward the Adam's apple (anterior displacement); it may be too far to the left or right (lateral displacement); it may be protruding more than the others (posterior displacement). By pulling a vertebra askew, as by tightening his shoulders, the person blocks the Energy channel between torso and head and traps his feelings inside the body below.

A displaced vertebra in the person's neck can sometimes be adjusted by simply holding your fingers directly over the bone and flowing Energy into the tension area. The body wants to return to its position of optimum functioning—the vertebra wants to return home—but an ego energy is holding the muscles connected to it in contraction. By flowing Energy under the principle of general transference, you help the muscles loosen so that the bone can spring back into place.

When it does, the energy below the block that has been pressuring for release comes surging forth. And there you have the second principle: energy can be released by correcting the body's structure.

Second Principle: Structural Correction

Here are more explicit instructions.

Suppose you're working on a person with a neck vertebra too far forward. Place a folded towel under his head to make the neck-line straighter. Surround the displaced vertebra with your fingers for a very long time—perhaps two or three minutes—or until you feel the energy waking up and moving into your body. His neck will begin to stretch by itself, making more space for the bone and opening a channel through which energy can flow upward.

To give an example: Daniel's body was quite rigid when he first lay down on the table. I massaged his chest but couldn't get any Energy flowing. I searched the shoulder and neck area: there was a gap in his spine where the fourth cervical vertebra should have been. So, after loosening his neck muscles generally, I held my palms under his head and reached with my index and middle fingers far into the neck to contact the buried vertebra. Two or three minutes went by, and finally a flow of energy began. His neck lengthened; the vertebra moved into line; and then Daniel began to moan. The sound—soft, desperate, resigned—came from deep within and was highly charged with energy. It seemed like the moaning went on forever, intense, charged, but never loud. His body began to tremble, while rushes of energy pushed upward through his head and out through me. I was tingling all over. When the stream finally subsided, Daniel was much more relaxed, and jubilant.

Structural displacement is always a signal that energy is trapped: the person has changed his physical organization to keep his feelings inside. When you see shoulders that are pinched in, a chest that is depressed, a hip that is too high, a pelvis that is too narrow, legs that are turned out, heels that are turned in, toes that are pulled up, you can expect to find imprisoned energies.

If a particular part of the body is out of place, you should flow in Energy there while you imagine—with the power of your center—the bones and tissues resuming their natural relationships with one another. This often helps the area to loosen its structural anomalies so that the bound energies may escape.

Take the case of pinched-in shoulders. Observing the person from behind, you would see his shoulder blades almost touching his spine and know that he ought to have more room in his thoracic cavity.

Have the person lie on his back while you face his right arm. Hold the upper arm with your left hand, the forearm or elbow with your right hand. Do not pull. Simply flow Energy into the arm, directing it toward the upper spine. When it reaches those tight muscles underneath the shoulder blade and near the spine, it activates the caught energies there. The area begins to expand, the person's arm floats outward by itself, and energies start zinging out through his arm, as well as his head and feet.

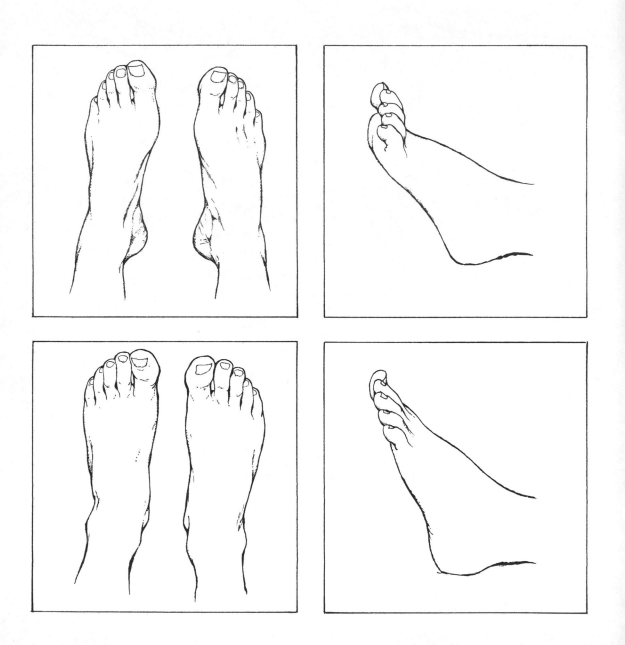

Another important place where a person typically breaks his flow structurally is at the feet. He may do this by turning in his heels, or by pulling up his toes.

He can distort his feet in either or both ways for various reasons. If the person has rejected his earth-nature, he is preventing Energy from traveling upward out of the earth into his body. If he has sent unwanted feelings as far away from his head or conscious mind as possible, he has buried energies in his feet. If he's holding qualities in the torso that he's not yet ready to lose, he's preventing energies from traveling into the ground. In any case, he pays the price of being physically and mentally ungrounded. He has lost his moorings, is given to instability. His body's natural balance—between earth and sky, between yin and yang—is disrupted.

When you are aligning a heel, you'll want the person lying on his back. After you have massaged the entire leg, cup both hands under the ankle. Flow Energy into the leg, all the way to the hip joint if possible. Then, gently pull the heel straight out, using your body as a weight. Returning to the ankle, press it sideways until the heel is exactly in line with the foot. Hold for at least ten breaths, to allow time for the person's Energy to pass through his ankle and out his foot.

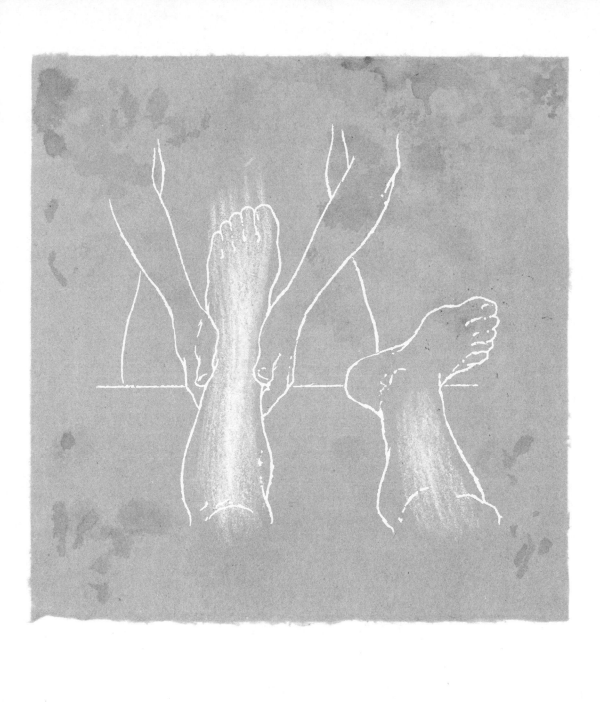

This technique helped one woman to unload the grief of a miscarriage.

I was massaging her overly thin, tight back when I happened to notice that both of her heels turned inwards at a forty-five degree angle to her legs. I had a sense of the energy in her back trying to release through the legs but being stopped at her ankles.

I asked her to turn over onto her backside. I pulled out her heels and straightened them little by little. An energy began to flow out. It was grief: she wailed in anguish over the loss of a child the year before. In ten minutes that was over, and the woman felt better than she had since the miscarriage.

When the person's toes are raised, rather than extending directly in line with the ball of the foot, you can expect energy locked in underneath the base of the toes, or sometimes in between them. The energy may be trying to leave the torso, using the legs as an escape route, but it is stopped by the last possible barrier.

To open the toes, massage the foot as suggested on page 62. Work the toes very thoroughly. Rotate them clockwise and counterclockwise. Pull them gently, always flowing Energy. Then kneel and press the ball of the foot flat with your thumbs. Push your thumbs upward under and between the toes, concentrating on raised toes, or hold the toes individually, until you find a spot where caught energy releases into you. Hold and breathe, and let the releasing energy travel through your body and aura into the ground.

Sometimes the toes are the only place you can reach the person. I smile when I think of the well-built 6'4", 200-pound Canadian farmer who remained unresponsive until I massaged the smallest toe on his left foot. I felt energy trying to come out there, so I stayed several moments until what felt like a lightning bolt zig-zagged down from his chest, across his belly to the hip joint, and out through his leg. He began to whimper sadly. It happened that his father had limped on his left leg, and in an attempt to love, or relate to his father, this man had developed a sympathetic limp as a child.

Wherever you are working—feet, hips, shoulders, neck, spine—
you will, hopefully, feel Energy or energies coming in to you from
the body.

Now, add another dimension to your awareness. With your eyes
closed, try to see how far the rays from your hands are traveling
into the body. Try to see where the energies traveling into you
are coming from. This is not really difficult. Almost anyone can
do it with a little practice, if not on the first try.

Third Principle: Seeing

You can see with the same inner faculty that feels Energy—your center. Your center is sensitive to light, a special luminescence that belongs to the flow. Seeing is a kind of feeling: feeling how a body is flowing inside. But in seeing, this knowledge takes on form, pattern, and dimension, qualities we usually associate with visual experience.

When you see a healthy body, you observe an inner radiance that emanates from center and flows out the feet, arms, head. When you see a body that is unhealthy, deadened by caught energies, you observe dark places or limbs that are not energized. If the caught energies are activated but have not yet moved out of the body, you will see a charge building up somewhere on the skin surface—for example, you may see heart feelings on their way out the arm gathered at the little finger.

Once you've seen the lines of Energy moving through a healthy body, you'll sense immediately when they are missing. You'll also know when they've been restored. So it is through seeing that you find out what corrections in the Energy flow are necessary.

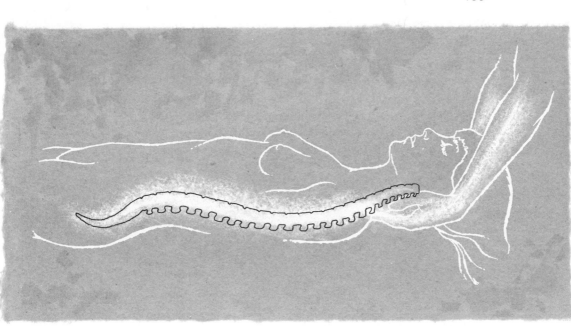

The easiest place to practice seeing is at the top of the person's spine. Try resting your hands on the seventh cervical vertebra, protruding at the base of the neck. Then close your eyes. Look out through your center. You will see an illumined line along the spinal column or a more diffused area of light that extends downward from your hands, perhaps three inches, perhaps to the waist, perhaps to the coccyx, perhaps all the way to the toes and beyond.

Now, suppose you are holding your hands at the top of the person's spine, and, with your eyes-closed vision, you see light filling up his torso, but nothing lower—the body appears to have no legs. Their absence signifies that they are blocked and need attention.

In this situation there are at least four things you can do.

First, you can massage the legs very carefully, using the principle of general transference. Look for a spot where jammed-up energy could escape if you were there to let it out and ground it. Such a spot, probably less than an inch in diameter, will give off more energy than surrounding skin surfaces.

Its location varies from person to person. Sometimes you can see it as a dark pressure point, sometimes you must simply be sensitive to the degree of flow under your hands. Let them be guided.

A second technique for moving blocked energy is to place your hands a certain distance from where the flow *is* and draw it toward the place where it *is not*. Suppose the person's Energy comes down through his leg to his knee, but no further. Place your hands where the Energy is coming out, in this case, at the knee. Then, move both hands several inches down the calf. Draw the person's Energy to your hands, and thus move the blocked energy that gets in its way, which may then pass out through you. Once contact with the flow is made again, move your hands down several inches more. Repeat this until you are beyond the foot and into the aura. Then the whole leg will be energized.

The third thing you can do when you see a blocked area in the body is to enclose that area with your hands and create a magnetic field between them.

Again, let's use the leg as an example. Place one hand above the block, where there is already a flow—over the groin or at the base of the spine. Place your other hand below the block—under the foot. Then breathe Energy into your hands. You will recall that your right hand is positive, your left negative; as they become energized by your breath, a magnetic field builds up. Once you have magnetic attraction, you can send Energy from one hand to the other, energizing the leg.

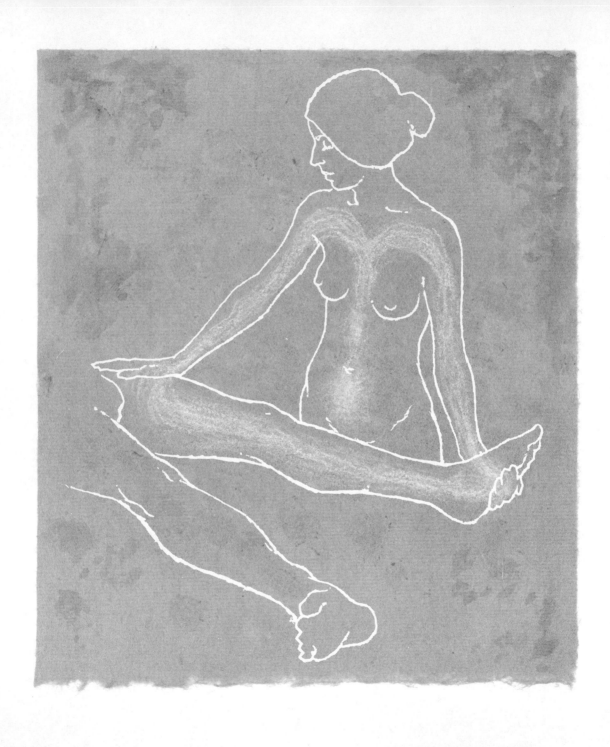

I used this technique when my friend Ian came to me for help. He'd broken his left elbow some months before, but when it healed he didn't regain his normal freedom of movement.

First, as usual, I worked on his shoulders and neck. I could see that Energy wasn't moving properly through his arm. Rather than being stopped at the elbow, however, it was blocked in the shoulder joint. So I held his left forearm with my left hand and his shoulder with my right, making contact with the Energy in his back. Soon I began to feel Energy filtering down through his arm into my left hand. He could feel it too. Tears of sadness drifted down his cheeks as I massaged the outside of the shoulder, then the upper arm. I moved my left hand to his fingers, so that the entire limb would be energized.

Afterwards, Ian told me that when he shifted his attention from his elbow to his shoulder, he remembered an incident in the hospital. His wife had visited: "She just looked at me—didn't reach out to touch me or do anything." By reliving the experience again, this time feeling his hurt and sadness, he released the blocked energy that had prevented movement in his arm.

With another woman, I saw that her right arm was flowing Energy, but her right hand was not. So I created a magnetic field between her forearm and her fingertips, using focused breathing to make the field stronger. After a minute or so, she broke into hysterical sobbing. Her mother had often slapped her irrationally as a child, and she had vowed she'd never be like her mother. Then, one day in a fit of anger, she slapped her own daughter. Horrified, she "cut off" her hand.

A fourth way of dealing with blocked energy is more difficult. You must send your own rays of light through the darkness. You do this through the power of mind. As you send out Energy (on the exhale), make a mental picture of the body having the flow that would make it healthy. Instead of keeping this imaginary picture in your brain, send it out through your center so that it's placed inside the body you're working on.

I decided to work with Irene in front of a group of people who were learning to see Energy. When I touched the top of her spine, I was dismayed to find no Energy flowing in her back. How could the group see what wasn't there? What should I do?

First, I asked another group member, Ken, to hold her feet. Then I placed my fingers over the second dorsal vertebra and imagined that there was a stream of light running down the length of Irene's spine to the coccyx. I concentrated very hard on this image, but not just with my head—my whole body, particularly the solar plexus, was involved in giving that idea power so that it would become a reality. I felt that my center actually included Irene's spine and it could therefore manifest the flow there.

Soon it began to happen. Energy began to move from my hands to her pelvis—the major work had been done. Now, I hoped the magnetic field between Ken and myself would activate a flow in her legs as well. It took about two minutes for the Energy to extend itself into her left leg, another minute to move into her right leg. Ken could feel it. The group could see it. Soon Irene was trembling, as the fear which had been blocked in her body began to exit through opened channels.

The technique of seeing applies to the auric bodies as well as the physical. You will have an eyes-closed sense of where Energy is or isn't balanced at some distance from the body.

To prepare for auric seeing, actually pass your hands over the person's front side from head to foot, about three or four inches from the body. Note the places where you feel a smooth, joyous current coming out from the person; these are balanced. Note the places where you feel jerky violent flows, or emotions that aren't moving, or dead, cold, empty space; these are imbalanced.

Now, stand at the person's head. With your eyes closed, look out of your center. You will see the very same balances and imbalances in the aura that you just felt with your hands. Give yourself time; the experience is subtle.

Once you trust your ability to see the aura, you will begin to notice that energies can be trapped there as well as in the body. They appear as dark spots, which are charged and therefore attract your attention. Sometimes they are as much as two feet away from the body, so you have to be sensitive and watchful. When you find such a spot, touch it with both hands (in the air, so to speak), and the energy may discharge through you. This restores balance to the aura, and ultimately to the body, which depends on the aura for its supply of life Energy.

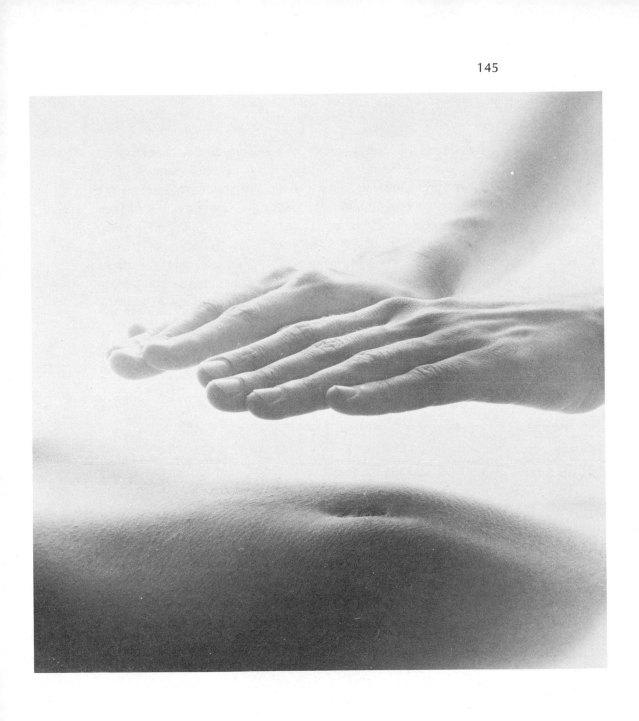

Sometimes you will contact an energy inside the body from a point outside the body. Suppose you lay your palms over a blocked area, and you find yourself unable to activate the energy there; however, you feel a shimmering above the backs of your hands. Unbalanced energy has gathered in the aura and is trying to tell you, "Work here." Raise your hands to that spot—usually three or four inches from the body. Inevitably, this will trigger physical release via unseen magnetic connections. The person may begin to vibrate, to shudder, to cry, as the energy in his body makes way for new life.

Through seeing the energy patterns in the body as a whole, you'll devise endless techniques for facilitating Energy flow.

Now that you've experimented with general transference, with structural correction, and with seeing, the fourth basic technique —psychic reading—should be easy. Already you've discovered the existence of energies: limited, definitive forms of life that have been locked into the person's psyche. Now you simply allow yourself to feel their qualities and to intuit the ways in which the person has defined or limited himself.

You will not clearly understand this until it happens for you. At some appropriate moment, you may be working with a body's energy and suddenly find yourself aware of more than tingling or flowing sensations. You may find yourself thinking: "This energy feels like I feel when I'm afraid . . . This energy has a fearful quality . . . This energy is fear."

Identifying the quality or the meaning of an energy is the essence of psychic reading.

Psychic reading, as you may have noticed, has to do with energies, rather than Energy. It has to do with the person's limitations, with the definitive aspects of his ego. It isolates the parts of a person that need to be balanced.

When you read, your job is to reintegrate those energies into the person's total flow.

Fourth Principle: Psychic Reading

Using your psychic ability for healing, for re-integration, is a task that requires sensitivity, tact, and caring. When you read for a person, you'll not only tell him of his qualities, but also of what he could do to make changes for health—if he's carrying sadness, for instance, he could cry. For this reason, you'll try to tune into him as a whole before you say anything. Look for the best way to present the information so that he can willingly receive it and be helped by it.

Above all, this demands a non-judgmental attitude. You must temporarily suspend your own morality, leave right and wrong behind, keep your vision of what *is* unclouded by concepts of what *should be*. When you affirm the way he is, you give the person the Energy he needs to cry, to shake, to allow the energies he's holding to move toward balance. Think of the person as being just the way he needs to be to take the next step in his own growth.

The best place to practice psychic reading is the spine. Have the person lie on his stomach. First, loosen the back generally with Energy massage (see pages 69–74). When you come to the point of massaging the vertebrae individually as you travel up the spine, check each vertebra for:

    structural position
    energy connection with vertebrae above and below
    strength of energy flow
    quality of energy flow

To try reading for the first time, you will want to locate vertebrae that are ready to reveal a specific energy content. Either these carry a strong unique vibration—spiraling, zizzing, undulating, pulsating rhythmically or arhythmically—or they are displaced. Displacement indicates an energy blockage, and your hands may offer the charge needed to clear it.

So now, having made initial exploration over the spine seeking vertebrae to read, pick an appropriate one, and hold your fingers on top of it for a minute or so. As you exhale, send Energy to the person at this location. As you inhale, take his energy into your center. Feel it.

To identify the quality of the energy you feel coming from this particular vertebra, pass it upward from your center to your head. Your head simply analyzes what your belly has already experienced. It categorizes the feeling, giving it a name: fear, indifference, satisfaction.

Most of the time you probably use your head differently. You organize the stimuli received from your sense organs according to concepts, and then you respond, or react emotionally, to your own conceptualization. The psychic function reverses the roles of the head and belly. First you feel with your belly. By the time the information gets to your brain, your emotional response is already completed. So your brain serves your center in an advisory capacity rather than a controlling one.

To read the energy clearly, you must be blank or empty inside your body. The blankness I'm talking about is a state of Energy awareness. There is flow and pulsation, but it is smooth, clear, pure, joyous, receptive, full—yet open and blank. Blankness in this sense does not mean a lack of feeling, like deadness or nothingness in the belly, which are ego energies. Rather, you are aware of the life-force; it becomes a backdrop for the more limited positive and negative qualities that come from the person's spine.

After you read one vertebra, move on to the next one that is ready. Generally, you should be moving up the spine. Wherever you read, though, make sure you flow in Energy at the same time to loosen the energy at that place. This gives the person a better chance of feeling it while the information is being given. Then, when you are finished, place your left hand at the base of the person's spine, your right hand over his neck or head, and pass Energy up the spine, between your hands, to connect the pieces you have explored separately.

You've used the spine to practice psychic reading because the vertebrae carry the energies of associated body parts; thus, each vertebra usually delineates a different, specific, and precisely defined energy. However, the same psychic principles apply elsewhere on the body. Wherever you happen to be massaging, listen with your belly for remarkable feelings, and then let them travel to your head for identification.

The information coming into your head from your belly will be categorized in several ways. I will discuss three and illustrate their use in healing.

First, you may directly identify an emotion or thought because you know how it feels in yourself. By telling the person he is sad in a certain part of his body, you may help make a connection between his head (conscious experience) and his body (subconscious experience) that he previously could not make for himself. Then, as you activate that part with Energy, he is able to feel his sadness, perhaps letting the caught energy disperse directly from its location or indirectly through tears and sounds.

If you are able to isolate the quality of the energy, but you can't recognize it by name, ask the silent question, "What is this?" An answer always comes to you. Usually it's the first word that enters your mind.

At first, ask the person about your interpretation. Find out whether he feels the same thing you do at a given place. If the person weeps when you tell him of his sadness, this is affirmation. Then, once you've learned what a certain energy—sadness— feels like, you will always recognize it. In time you won't have to ask if your reading is correct; you'll know.

A second way to identify energy psychically is through mental pictures or visions. These pictures may be visually distinct, as in a dream, but more often they are feelings, or shadow-like forms, of a situation. For instance, you may feel how the person, as a child, experienced his mother: she required so smoothly and graciously that he conform to proprieties that he didn't realize he was being manipulated. Again, because you are in a blank state, you know these feeling-pictures represent the quality of that person's energy.

These pictures may have literal or symbolic meaning.

An example of a vision to be interpreted literally would be seeing a person's dog hurt when the person was five years old. Here is a situation that has actually happened—and the person, perhaps, is still holding grief connected with the experience.

An example of a vision to be interpreted symbolically would be a flying bird. This is a symbol I often experience to mean the person is ungrounded, or not well integrated with his physical existence.

Symbols have to be interpreted within the context of feeling. For example, a flying bird may not always indicate a lack of earthiness. If the bird feels hawk-like, it may mean simply that one part of the person is preying on another part.

Symbol systems are unique to each individual; your images mean certain things only to you, mine only to me. The same information that comes to me in the form of a flying bird may come to you in the form of a spaceship.

There may also be pictures of past eras, where the clothes, life-styles, environment will belong to other centuries and locations. These can be explained in terms of reincarnation. Or, they can be treated simply as literal/symbolic. The important thing is that they represent bound-up energy, which the person can release if he is willing to experience its particular quality in himself.*

*See Appendix A, example one.

Besides feeling and seeing, you may develop a third psychic ability: hearing. If the energy trapped in a body wants release vocally, you may hear words or sentences the body needs to say, sounds the body needs to make.

If you hear words, they will often be charged verbatim. Other words expressing the same idea won't do, because the energy is attached to the exact phrase as yet unsaid. Sometimes the words will be in a foreign language: "no" won't work when "nyet" is required. For one woman I worked on, the word "God" in English had no meaning, yet the word "Gott" in Danish was highly charged.

If you hear words psychically, ask the person to say them at least three times, pausing between each repetition. This gives his intellect and his feelings a chance to connect. Ask the person to listen inwardly to whether the sentence fits his bodily experience.

As with words, a person may have withheld a sound at a time it needed expression—for example, a woman laboring to bear a child, this lifetime or some other. If you hear a sound, make the sound aloud as an example which the person can imitate.

The sounds that need to be made are not necessarily withheld sounds. Often, they are required because they resonate the flesh in a way that would open it. For instance, you'll hear a high *eee* sound in a body which needs opening in the top of the head. A very nasal *ong* or *nong* sound will free the nasal cavities and upper-front of the head. In general, the sounds required range from *O* to *ahh* to *eee* as you move up the torso from belly to head.

You should never ask a person to make a sound on the basis of an intellectual decision, but rather on the basis of a psychically intuited need. Otherwise, the sound releases no energy and is a waste of time.

Another interesting thing about sounds is that often you are able to provide them when the person cannot. You can sing into the person's spine; you will actually feel the body resonate when you hit the right vowel and pitch.

Occasionally, it happens that you can become a channel for speech as well as sounds. An interesting example of this involved a woman who could not connect her voice with her belly, even though the words "I'm dying" were the right ones. So I suggested that I try being the voice for her belly. I said several short sentences which seemed to pass from her belly out through me. It worked. The compacted vibrations broke loose and we felt them shivering our auras. Then, the woman remembered that she had almost died of pneumonia some months after she was born. That explained why the words didn't link up energetically—she didn't have them at the time.

V

The Psyche Viewed Psychically

So that you will have some idea what kind of things may be intuited psychically, I'd like to sketch some of the more typical psychological patterns I pick up in people's bodies. These are:

     win-loss
     death
     masculine/feminine imbalance
     helplessness
     misinterpretation of feeling
     fantasy

By far the most common is the win-loss syndrome. In this condition, the person lives under the shadow of his own conceptual ideals; he carries ideas of what is right, or perfect, and wrong, or imperfect. If he fulfills his ideals, he wins; if he doesn't fulfill his ideals, he loses.

The person judges himself according to concepts he has constructed. Yet, often he doesn't realize he's doing this because he projects the judge-role onto a parent or teacher or friend or society in general.

To understand projection, you must accept the principle that a person's environment is created by his internal reality. His outside world is determined by his inside world. The various energies he holds attract people with compatible or sympathetic vibrations, and they become appropriate mirrors for his own ego qualities. So, when he thinks he is reacting to someone out there, he is really reacting to an energy carried in his own body.

In the case of a win-loss pattern, the person may project the judge and be the defendant. If he is judged (by himself) to be wrong, he experiences a loss.

When the person loses (according to his own standards) he feels pain, resentment, anger, fear, hostility, sadness. If these responses are unacceptable to him, he controls himself, or his environment, to prevent himself from experiencing them.

Control, or manipulation, always indicates a win-loss pattern. A person controls to make right or good things happen and to prevent wrong or bad things from happening.

This person no longer trusts the flow. "Unless I control," the feeling goes, "things will turn out wrong and I will lose." Inevitably the person has *already experienced* the very loss he is protecting himself from. He retained his previous hurt or grief by not letting himself feel it at the time. Since the Energy which surrounds him has a natural tendency toward balance, it is always pushing him into similar loss situations so that the held energy might be reactivated. If the person doesn't understand what's happening, he keeps protecting himself from the repeated losses. He refuses to let them happen, he tries to control. His body becomes rigid and inflexible as more and more losses, which he refuses to feel, are stopped inside. Understandably the world begins to look antagonistic to him.

If, however, the person comes to understand what's happening, he is no longer threatened by the outer stimuli. Rather, he uses them to activate the feelings—the pain, the sadness—that need to be discharged.

A person can transcend the win-loss syndrome by understanding that in Energy there is no winning or losing, no good or bad. Good and bad are value judgments based on mental concepts or ideas of how things should be, as opposed to how they are. Concepts have no life. When a person gives up his reverence for these concepts, when he takes back his power to do what he wants to do, rather than what he thinks he ought to do, he can move in the direction of a more fluid, satisfying existence.

Interestingly enough, the person may see that he is living for an image he has of himself, or a plan of how he should be, and he may be unwilling to change. He is accustomed to his ego identity. He feels he exists because he is heavy, static, stable, predictable, solid, immovable. He prefers this to being unstable, moving, flowing, ecstatic, joyful—in short, alive.

It may then be a matter of re-educating the person regarding the nature of death.

Death is a paradox:
   The only real death is ego.
   Death of ego brings en-lightened-ment.
   There is no death.
These contradictory statements are all true, but each requires a different interpretation of the word death.

THE ONLY REAL DEATH IS EGO.

Ego energies, held energies, prevent life from flowing in a body. Therefore, they create a feeling of hardness, a lack of mobility, a static condition. This is death. This is an existence where Energy and vitality have been replaced by lethargy and depression.

Nevertheless, the person who carries ego energies begins to feel that they *are* himself. At least he has, or holds, something inside. No one can take that away from him. In other words, he becomes attached to the energies. To give them up would be to lose himself, to die.

DEATH OF EGO BRINGS EN-LIGHTENED-MENT.

The second meaning of the word death refers to giving up held energies. This can be very frightening for a person who is attached to them. There is a loss involved. He will have to empty the spaces which are presently filled with energies like sadness, pain, or helplessness. That requires a great risk on his part. What if nothing fills the empty space?

To die in this second sense requires the faith that wherever an energy flows out, Energy flows in. In short, it requires trust. And that trust is rewarded, sometimes quickly, sometimes over a longer term, by changes in the person that could be described as lightness. The person becomes less weighty, less emotionally heavy. His walk is more springy, he feels buoyant and floating—high—most of the time. He looks and feels radiant, glowing, shining. The light inside him has been turned on.

This kind of death is not easy. There is always pain involved, as one lets go of something he thought was himself.

Paul carried male supremacy energy in his right shoulder, just under the collar bone. To integrate his right and left sides, he would have to give it up. He understood that it would be painful to lose the identity he had always known.

Nevertheless, he decided to take a risk. As I held my hands over that place, he began to whimper, then to sob gently. Just as he experienced the emotional pain of ripping the ego in his right shoulder, a rush of love came from his left side, and his feminine and masculine aspects were joined. The difference in the Energy level was incredible: he was at least four times more alive. I, too, found myself crying, saddened by the thought that people could choose ego over Energy, when Energy was so much more nourishing.

THERE IS NO DEATH.

This refers to physical death. Physical death is merely the juncture at which the person leaves behind the physical vehicle he has used on the earth plane. After death, he still experiences the Energy he knew at this level.

If a person is afraid of death, it is because he has associated physical death with the loss of his ego-self or his deadness, in the first sense of the word. In a way, this is justified because his ego energy exists in time—with a beginning, a middle, an end. It has a death. However, when it ends, a person comes to experience a reality which is endless, timeless, and has no limits. Then, and only then, does the person realize that death is not real.*

*See Appendix A, example two

The third psychological problem which is common in my readings is masculine/feminine imbalance.*

Every body is bi-polar; it contains both masculine and feminine aspects. The body is in balance sexually when the masculine gives to the feminine, and the feminine receives from the masculine; the positive feeds the negative, creating movement toward equilibrium. If the exchange between the two is interrupted, the body is literally immobilized to some degree.

*See Appendix A, examples three and four.

Take, for example, the man in whom I saw a wolf symbolizing his masculine energy (right side) and a sheep symbolizing his feminine (left side). The wolf was hungry. I could see him prowling on a bleak, barren landscape, yellow with dust because there was no water to support vegetation and other animals. I imagined he would gobble up whatever living thing came his way. The sheep I experienced as gentle, sensitive, and very frightened of being nibbled, eaten, or devoured. It was clear to me that when this man's masculine energy approached his feminine, the female in him would run. And this was an ongoing pattern.

Two things would help this man break his pattern. One, he must understand the feminine fear as the ego fear of losing self. Self is never lost, only fear is lost, which the person mistakenly thinks is himself. If that fear were "eaten," it might be a pleasant experience in which withheld energy would be discharged and vital Energy restored.

Two, he must realize that he created the wolf's environment. He created it as unnourishing because he wanted it that way: not getting what he needed was a very skillful method of keeping himself immobilized. To move toward sexual balance, this man must change the wolf's environment to a fertile earth where he can have more than his fill of good things—full-fill-ment.

A person's masculine and feminine aspects have definite personalities. These two personalities may be loving one another, in which case they are balanced. Or they may be fighting one another, in which case they are unbalanced. In the latter case, they are *polarized*. The male separated from the female becomes very yang, very positively charged, very aggressive. Likewise, the female separated from the male becomes very yin, very negatively charged, very withdrawn and protective.

Sandra's body exhibited these polarizations. Her female aspect, located in the aura above her head, was characterized by the word purity. Her male aspect, pushing up through her torso, felt devilish. The feminine part didn't want to let the devil in for fear of losing a quality which was precious to her. The devil, on the other hand, became more insidious the longer he was kept out. Sandra described this as "my tail getting sharper."

During a session, in a moment of trust Sandra opened her purity space to her devil. She was amazed by what happened. The devil, who had been so pushy and pointed, became the agent of pleasure. He mellowed and treated her gently. The female aspect reported warm, good sensations. But then she got scared of the feelings and closed up again. Immediately the devil returned to his harsh manners.

Sandra's case offers a general procedure you can use in dealing with masculine/feminine imbalance. First, define the polarities. This is where psychic ability is especially valuable. You'll want to identify in detail the energies of the two sexual aspects, usually carried in the right and left halves of the person's body, so that he gets in touch with them experientially. Particularly with men, help them feel the female inside who may be saying, "Sex is wrong, and I don't want to be wrong," or "I never get what I need." Common polarizations are listed on the next page, but it's important that you intuit the person's qualities exactly, rather than working from generalizations.

Examples of
Polarized Qualities

A	B
distant	lonely
controlling	defensive
dominant	helpless
	lacking allies
superior	inferior
stable	dissatisfied
immovable	
proud	resigned
hateful	hated
disdainful	rejected
killer	fearful
	pleading
	("Don't kill me")
	defiant
	("I won't let
	you kill me")

Categories A and B may apply to either the masculine or the feminine aspect, or they may represent some kind of split other than sexual.

Then, help the person to understand that when these polarized qualities are brought together, they change. The devil mellows. Purity feels pleasure. The killer gives life. The killed is resurrected. Separated, the opposites appear to be untrustworthy, but when let out of their cages, they join the mainstream of love and become valuable resources.

The fourth psychological problem I'd like to discuss is helplessness. Helplessness can be confusing because a person tends not to take responsibility for it. He will draw your pity and your sympathy, rather than your assistance in making a change. Avoid this trap by understanding how helplessness works.

Helplessness is a choice. And it is always held in relation to its opposite polarization—coercion or domination or control—also contained in the same body. When the person experiences helplessness being forced on him by his environment, it is because he's projected the authority figure in himself outward. He is threatened by a power he doesn't realize is his own.

Once the person understands, or experientially verifies, these two parts of himself, he finds out that helplessness is not real, but rather his own creation. He can change that creation by assuming power—the ability to respond. Then the helpless energy isn't needed anymore and it tends to discharge. He can facilitate that release by feeling helpless fear, letting it flow over his body, and by making sounds like "Help." Often, he relives a key experience from the past in which he felt helpless.

However, it may also happen that when the person feels his helplessness, it doesn't flow out. This means that the person, at this time, is unwilling to change. He is acting out the energy rather than discharging it. If you ask him to feel as helpless as possible and then to tell you what he's getting from being that way, his answers will be something like this:

"I can manipulate other people into giving me love and attention."

"I don't have to be responsible for my actions, or feelings like anger and hostility."

"I prefer to be dominated, to play the inferior role."

The person also gets the helplessness itself. He feels enlivened, so to speak, by that specific quality of energy. Once he realizes that he *wants* this particular energy, that he *likes* how it charges him, or at least that he's used to it, he has the chance to make a choice between this limited energy and the larger Energy.

Two other psychological conditions can be helped particularly by psychic intuition. Therefore, I mention them here, even though they are less common than the previous four.

First, a person may misconstrue the meaning of an energy in his body. For example, he may have sexual feelings that he misinterprets as anger; or angry feelings that he takes to be sexual. If his sadness, pain, disappointment energies rigidify his body, he may perceive them incorrectly as strength. By trusting your psychic sense, you can help him to clear up this confusion. Usually the person is greatly relieved when he learns what his feeling really is—now he can deal with it appropriately.

In the second condition, the person carries fantasy energy. Fantasy is a quality of energy comparable to helplessness, hostility, etc. It feels like the person is saying, "Let's pretend," or "Isn't it beautiful in this other world."

Some people like this quality of energy, perhaps because they think it's safe. I have worked with people who imagined killing their mother or making love with their dream woman, yet the energy coming from their bodies was not remotely connected with hatred or with sex. It was fantasy energy. This is an important realization if the goal is to work for energy release, and the energy won't release until the person experiences its quality exactly.

To close, here's an account of a complete two-hour session, so you'll get an idea of what is possible with psychic massage.

It was the first time I had worked with Edward. He had had some group therapy before, but he had never experienced a massage, nor had he worked with Energy as such.

I began, as in a typical massage, working on his chest. Immediately, I felt sadness coming from his heart. Concentrating there for several minutes, I saw an overlay of lonely images from his time in the Armed Services, but I felt the sadness had evolved previously and that it was connected with his mother. "She was committed [to a mental institution] when I was thirteen and died when I was twenty-one," he responded to my queries. "I remember feeling I couldn't hold us both up. She died that I might live —and there was nothing I could do." By this time he was weeping, but there was no energy release; instead, his tears seemed to be holding something in. When a person tells me there was nothing he could do, he has usually overlooked the one change he could make: release of feeling in himself. So I was looking for that, particularly in the projected role. I explained to Ed, "You are your mother . . . the physical world is an illusion in that the pieces you see are yourself projected . . . you must reown the part represented by your mother." I asked him to change his original sentence around to "I died that you might live," and this time his crying was real—energy-laden.

Next I was drawn to his left foot. The energy there had the quality of distance. I saw an image of Ed on a ship; land was far away.

I interpreted the symbolism to mean that Ed experienced distance from his physical nature. He was floating, away from his body, out of touch with reality. In order to reverse his pattern, I asked Ed to try a sentence which was opposite to the symbolic message: "I contain all things in my body." Naturally, he balked at the reference to things. So I pushed him further with the sentence "I am a thing: my body." Again, he resisted, until he remembered some of the catechism of his Christian Science upbringing: "Spirit is real, the body is unreal, a 'mortal error'." As he said the words, he exuded heavy energy discharge. Afterwards, we discussed briefly a new understanding of the body as spirit made dense. Material things are not separate from God. They, too, are a vibration of the spirit.

Edward concluded: "I am all things," and paused. "But I am also nothing. How can that be?" He was confused and could not find an answer. I asked him to bring his awareness into his stomach while I held my hands two inches above. And he discovered the synthesis: "I am." Edward said, "I feel like a pillar. The feeling goes from top to bottom."

I was pleased. My goal was to energize his whole body, and we were well on our way. I could feel, however, that his head was not completely with the experience. So I moved my hands to his head to give the Energy that would help clear it. I instructed Ed about the two ways of using one's head: to control or to psychically identify what is. His head still wanted to control, and the sentence I heard it saying was, "I won't let go of my voice." Amidst tears, he began to let go of his voice by making a low sound, and that brought up a memory of his aunt and grandparents. "They won't hear me . . . If I speak loud, they'll go away. I'll speak low so they'll have to come close. But then they can't hear me . . ." Ed spoke in a tone of anguish. He asked me directly, "Can you hear me?" I replied, "Yes." He cried as a child cries.

Now, his head was open up to the temples but still blocked on top. In order to let Energy rise through that upper portion, I asked Ed to make an *eee* sound, rising from a soft low *eee* to a high loud scream. He protested that he'd tried it before, but it always came out phony. Under my insistence, he did it again—and it came out phony . . . no energy. But at least it gave me a chance to see psychically the reason he wouldn't let go of his voice completely. He used it to control people, especially himself; and giving up control would mean death. Ego would no longer exist. I asked Ed to alternate between the sentences, "I won't let go of control." "I'm willing to let go of control." At first, his sympathies were for the former, but after a moment he made a decision— to me astounding— in favor of the latter. A heavy fear began to rise up out of his abdomen. His body became contorted. Fear filled his head; but not enough of it could discharge. I suggested he release the energy in sounds. Finally, he allowed two short yelps, highly charged with very fast energy. He said the sounds were finished. But, no, I heard psychically sounds that were now angry, rather than fearful. "Get out." But he wouldn't say it loud. His voice was controlled; he would not give out the anger energy. Then, finally, it burst forth: "Get out and don't come back!"— and he cried sadness.

His next sentence was: "I don't have a place." This was compre-
hensible, since under the principle of projection, he had sent
himself away. "Where am I?" he called out. I suggested to him
the sentence: "I'm here."

"I'm here, I'm HERE!" he was crying with a heavy outpouring of
energy. It was real for him. I asked whether he was satisfied
where he was, and he answered, "Very."

VI

Postulates

Psychic massage is a system of healing. Like any other system it is built upon postulates—a set of presuppositions or proposed truths. Some of these are necessary for the system to work; others are helpful, but not necessary. First, let's examine the basic postulates which you must accept in order to do psychic massage.

1. Energy exists.
2. Energy flow is related to breath.
3. Energy circulates freely in a healthy body.
4. Attitudes or feelings can block Energy when their energy is separated, or withheld, from the total flow.
5. Withheld energies occupy space in the body at definite locations.
6. Withheld energies have qualities which can be psychically identified.
7. Withheld energies can be activated and moved by the application of Energy.

How can these postulates be verified?

Verification simply requires the phenomenological viewpoint that the feelings within your own body are real. Your body has receptors that give you access to information on many levels other than the physical. This can be known only by experience. Once you experience a past-life recall, for example, it's difficult to accept the idea that physical death is the end of existence. In short, if you have personal subjective experience, you don't need objective, intellectually determined conceptions to validate that experience for yourself. Instead, you will put the burden on your intellect to classify and organize subjective experience.

I believe that if you use this book as a guide, you will be able to experientially validate the premises of psychic massage for your-self.

There are other postulates that I personally believe will be helpful in your work, but they are not required. You may not experience these right away.

1. Energy is the substance of all things. It is available in unlimited supply.

2. There is no death, only departure from the physical plane or dimension of existence.

3. A person's physical body is the visible form of his auric bodies. It is his mind given density. Thus, the body is literally the shape of consciousness.

4. The body is a focusing mechanism, like a prism or a crystal. It channels Energy to make creative changes in the physical world.

5. Every person is totally responsible for his own personal universe. He attracts an environment that reflects his attitudes. He chooses conditions of childhood and adulthood.

6. The physical environment functions as a mirror or screen for projections. Although a person carries many energies in his body, he identifies with only a few. The others he projects onto the persons or conditions of his environment so that they are seen as outside.

7. The universe is in perfect order. Not a thing is out of place. From the viewpoint of karmic or cosmic equilibrium, there is a reason for every event.

8. Energy is another name for God.

9. Prayer works.

I would like to elaborate on these last two beliefs. You will remember that when I was discussing how Energy feels, I used the words:

> Love
> Light
> Acceptance (Grace)
> Perfection
> Peace
> Unending Now (Infinity)
> Patience
> Power to do good (Good will)

These are words people have been using for centuries to describe God. The more one's feelings are freed, the more one can feel being and the more one knows that God Is.

Prayer is atunement to that reality. "Not my will, but thine be done" is another way of saying, "I'm the only one who gets in the way of a truly harmonious existence." I find that praying while I work increases the amount of Energy available. In my experience, the most helpful things I can do to restore balance in someone's body are to thank God for the Energy to make the person well and to ask that nothing in my body or mind get in the way of the gift.

Given the preceding tenets, I'll add one more, which is my view of the nature of man.

10. Man is an entity created by God to know Him (LOVE), and to know harmony by experiencing self-chosen lack of harmony. His job is to build ego, then break ego; to learn control, then let go of control; to feel the reality of contained energies, but ultimately to enjoy the reality of a flow that washes through like a river and makes things right—perfect.

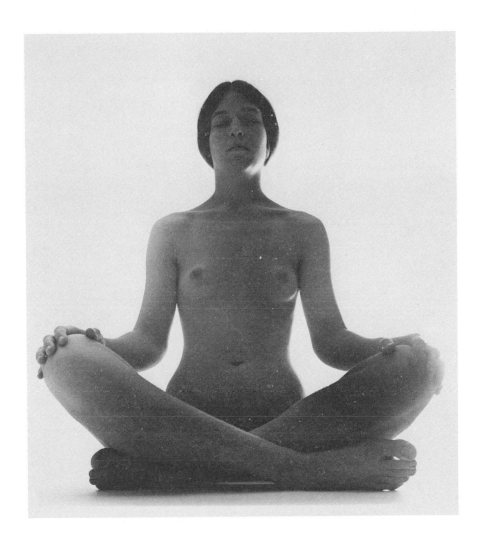

Appendix A: Past Life

So very often in my readings, I experience data that do not belong to the person's present existence. For instance, I may see the person on a ship with sails, obviously not in the twentieth century. Or, I may feel a quality that I know is ancient Egyptian, as with a priestess about to undergo initiation. I believe the explanation for these phenomena is reincarnation—that a person lives more than one lifetime. In the examples that follow, I will take this point of view.

EXAMPLE 1: DIANE

The first time I gave Diane a massage, I found protectiveness in her shoulders and saw psychically a chastity belt over her loins. From the vibrations, it was clear that she wouldn't let go of these qualities because she associated them with positive open feelings in her belly. She wouldn't be so free, were she not protected.

In the second session, I saw her in medieval France. That is to say, I saw her in a long dress overseeing the baking of bread in a castle kitchen. Her vibration felt aristocratic and unmistakably French. (To locate a place, I often visualize a map and find myself hovering over the right country as if it were a magnet.)

I experienced Diane holding energy related to her husband of that time. The relationship felt romantic—characterized by distance between the two—and her excitement derived from imaginative fantasies of her lover rather than any real connection with him. I was amazed by the fairy-tale quality of the situation.

Apparently her husband had ridden away, perhaps to war, and she awaited his return, wearing a chastity belt as a symbol of her affection for him. Diane was able to see the scene as well. "Either he never came back, or he came back unable to function as a male," she added from her own internal vision.

According to the cultural norms of that time, there was no way for her to take another mate. Diane described going to a nearby garden and seeing bright flowers, "like poppies," and telling herself not to cry, as it did not befit her station. I saw the flowers as a symbol of new life, Energy, that would have helped her to cry. Then Diane had a vision of herself sobbing somewhere, which was followed by a picture of an older woman, in the same garden, looking at a sundial and feeling "glad my misery will end soon." I asked her to backtrack a little, to become the younger woman, and to see if she could discharge the tears physically. Mental experience was not going to be enough. She was able to cry, though she continually expressed amazement at all her sadness. A sentence came with it: "I don't want to be alone."

After completing a session like this, a person usually sees ways in which the same energy is manifesting itself in the present. Diane was divorced, so being alone was the immediate reality of her existence. Also, she told me she had been interested in French Medieval poetry as long as she could remember, without knowing why.

The theory of reincarnation helps in dealing with a specific energy problem: fear of death. People die traumatically. Then they carry their fear of annihilation forever after. Often they must recall a particular death before the energy can be discharged.

EXAMPLE 2: MARK

In one session, I psychically saw my client as an old patrician in Rome: he was pleading, "Spare me." As he repeated the words aloud, he actually went back in time to that era and re-experienced the fear of impending execution. By the process of feeling it, he released his fear. Then, immediately following that discharge, I saw him in a Turkish war, at a time in his lives before the Roman incarnation. Sabers were flashing and somebody's head was being cut off. Then I saw it: "Mark, it was your head!" As he flashed back and re-experienced the scene, I saw it psychically through his eyes: the clamor, the confusion, a horse charging wildly by, and then a tremendous welling of fear. I screamed involuntarily, terrified. The energy of that sound seemed to come out of Mark through me. Afterwards, we were both shaking with the residue of the fear manifested by that sound.

Another problem better understood by a past-life viewpoint is masculine/feminine imbalance. Usually when I look psychically for the cause of a person's sexual problems, it is to be found prior to his childhood. The person already carried sexual polarizations before this birth. He chose parents and now chooses sexual partners, who are appropriate projection screens for his energies.

EXAMPLE 3: PHIL

Phil had lived previously as a Bedouin Arab. In that life, maleness was superior to femaleness. Females were property, like goats or other animals. Without conscious awareness, Phil created a pattern where his male aspect was positively valued and his female aspect was totally blocked. In his present life, Phil had a mother who indeed represented his feminine side: she was incapable of providing nourishment. While this enraged him, it was the inevitable result of a pattern started long ago.

Another way that male/female imbalance manifests itself karmi-cally is when the person becomes both of his aspects succes-sively, rather than merely projecting them. If a male has rejected females in one life, he may choose to be reborn as a female and experience being rejected—primarily because he carries both aspects within himself and each needs expression.

EXAMPLE 4: JULIE

I've worked with several women who I'm sure were men in other lifetimes. Julie particularly fascinated me in this respect. Although presently Caucasian, she had an Oriental past-life background. The words yin and yang designated her aspects much better than masculine and feminine. I saw that she had been a Japanese man of great personal power and strength, who had distanced himself from the feminine—his wife—and found his identity in business and intellect—the "superior" world. Now, as a female, Julie ex-perienced the helplessness, the despair, the loss in her feminine side. Because she knew no other alternative, she had held that pain under cover of resignation: "I'll just have to do it all myself."

Working with past-life energies has taught me that all experience is symbolic. The things that happen to us can be more usefully treated as symbols for our inner condition than as causally induced events explainable only in terms of space and time.

EXAMPLE 5: LINDA

In Linda's body, I saw a 12 year old girl sitting outside a one room cabin in Appalachia. She was undernourished, her bones protruding under a thin, torn dress. Her eyes looked scared and hopeless; she obviously had nothing. I asked Linda to experience the hunger feelings in her stomach and to give them verbal expression. The sentence "I'm empty" finally brought forth her tears, and much of the held loss energy was discharged.

Then, I glimpsed a life previous to the Appalachian one. The location was not given. All I saw was that her lover had just gone away. Because she had lost her center to him—he had been her center, her source—she was left with nothing. I knew psychically that she had later chosen the Appalachian setting to externalize her inner reality.

The symbolic nature of experience makes it unimportant whether you interpret past-life energy literally. The important thing is for the person to experience within himself the qualities associated with that particular caught energy (even if strange to this age). Once the energy discharges, he is that much more open to experience the present.

Appendix B: Cleansing

Working with energies sometimes has its problems. If you catch in your body the vibrations someone else is discarding, you can be affected by them afterwards, to the point of becoming ill. To avoid this, I always perform certain cleansing rituals when I massage.

Beforehand I
    spread balanced Energy throughout my workspace,
    pray that my body be protected from harmful influence—
        when the prayer works my auric glow, a tingling feeling,
        gets stronger.
During the massage I
    pass unbalanced energies through my legs into the earth,
    dip my hands into a nearby bowl of water if I suddenly feel
        dizzy, nauseous, or drained, because water absorbs toxins
        gathered in the aura.
Afterwards I
    always wash my hands,
    bathe, in epsom salts if possible,
    purify my massage room by burning 1 cup of epsom salts
        soaked in several tablespoons of alcohol,
    dismiss the person's work from my thoughts, because it is not
        mine.

Roberta DeLong Miller was born in Tacoma, Washington. She studied classi-
cal piano and viola for many years—and notes that many of the skills she
developed now apply to her massage work. She graduated from Carleton
College with a Philosophy major. Her interest in massage developed at the
Esalen Institute in Big Sur, California, where she worked for over two years,
heading the massage department for one year. There Roberta met and
married Dennis Miller, who designs and constructs massage tables. They
now reside in Boulder, Colorado. Roberta has taught massage in the United
States, Canada, and Europe and presently is developing a self-directed
method for integrating body and spirit.